IMPORTANT DISCLAIMER

In serious conditions like Crohn's, always seek medical advice from your Doctor. It is not the intention of this book to diagnose, prescribe, or replace medical care. This is not a medical book. The choices I have made may not work for you because we are all individuals. If you do anything that I have recommended, without the supervision of a licensed medical Doctor, you do so at your own risk. This information is provided with the hope that it may be helpful for those who choose to take greater responsibility for their own health.

Author: Tommi Sundqvist
The Naked Gut – true story
Self published 2018, Kaarina, Finland.
Translators: Liz Barrington and Eveliina Valkeapää
Proofreader: Janette St Pierre, Heli Mikkola
Pictures: Marko Airismeri, Heli Mikkola, Shutterstock
Text design and layout: Sanna Kostamo
EPUB/Kindle: Amie McCracken
ISBN 978-952-94-0842-9 (black and white)
ISBN 978-952-94-0843-6 (color version)
ISBN 978-952-94-0844-3 (e-book)
Global Register of Publishers
To contact the author, please send email to tommisun@gmail.com.
For more info: www.nakedgut.blogspot.com

"The book is very interesting and up-to-date because it refers to how the rate of intestinal diseases has exploded in recent years. It's also ingenious due to its versatility. This well-designed book is not just a reference to the intestines and illness, but it's a comprehensive piece of work that combines useful facts and great personal experience. It includes good treatment tips and nutritional information that's heartfelt and highly-supportive. In addition to providing health advice, the potential for financial savings to the patient and to the government are enormous. Oh, I wish people would understand what difference lifestyle and nutritional choices can make instead of them getting discouraged from what they could do to help themselves by simple changes in habits and responsibility. I'd definitely recommend this book to professionals too!"

*Anna Hämäläinen, Pharmacist, Finland*


"In the book you combined scientific research, well-documented resources and personal stories to back up your case for natural healing versus chemicals to "treat" IBS/IBD, Crohn's and ulcerative colitis. I liked the fact that you told your own personal story and then combined it with a healthy balance of nutrition, exercise, and your love of travel and meeting new people combined with the support from family an friends. The photos of your travels, your young adulthood, and inspirational pics from the photographer you worked with will be inspiring to all of those suffering from your disease. I really believe that your story will inspire and be a live-changing experience for millions of people that share your disease."

*Gene Casciari, USA*


"This book is a great example of body's intelligence and the power to restore itself to health, providing it is allowed to do so. It also empowers us to take the responsibility for our own health, as prevention is always preferable to cure. Thank you Tommi for sharing your incredible story with us."

*Päivi Jalasvirta, England Nutritional therapist, Dipl. CNM/London, LKL ry., RATY ry.*

THIS BOOK IS
DEDICATED TO THE
GUT ALMIGHTY

TRUST YOUR GUT
FEELING

# CONTENTS

**The Naked Gut – Introduction**   **6**
Foreword   8
Background: Tommi Sundqvist   9
I am forever grateful   10

**Why I chose my own path**   **12**
Gut bacteria is crucial in our life   14
Not knowing has forced me to
make difficult decisions   15
Digestive system – in a nutshell   17

**Three common digestive disorders:
IBS, IBD and Leaky Gut**   **21**
IBS – Irritable Bowel Syndrome   21
IBD – Inflammatory Bowel Disease   22
Leaky gut – The link to all
autoimmune diseases?   24
5 diagnoses to check   27
Autoimmune diseases are soaring   29

**My story**   **33**
Doctor's advice   36
3 wake-up calls   37
2 major surgeries in 7 days   41
MRSA   45
CAL-PRO – a test to detect
inflammation in the intestines   47
Colonoscopy   49
Goodbye medicine   51
And the healing started
– Recovery took 2 long years   52
Diet has a role in my recovery   55
Tommi's key points   56
Money and social security   58
Being healthy saves you
a fortune!   60

The way we live today   61
For the love of sports   64

**Travelling with IBD**   **66**
Florida – The sunshine state   67
Egypt - Land of Pharaoh's and
their revenge   69
Peru – The most magical place
in South America   72
Adventure in India   77
Greece – The land of gods and
goddesses   80
Handy all-around travel tips   82

**Tools for healing**   **86**
1. Mind   87
2. Detox   89
3. Individual diet – Find the least
harming food for you   93
About SCD[tm]   93
Avoiding harmful foods   96

**Different meal ideas**   **99**
Gut specific foods and recipies   102
Healthy oils   106
Healthy drinks   108
Supplements   109

**Another approach by functional
medicine**   **114**
Pasi Heinonen – story   118
Sanna Kostamo – story   119

**Sources**   **126**

# THE NAKED GUT – INTRODUCTION

Dear Reader,

This is a true story of a patient with one clear mission: To stay healthy and happy despite having a severe autoimmunity disease.

My name is Tommi Sundqvist, I'm 49 years old (born 1969). I am sharing my story as an inspiration to anyone who suffers from digestive disorders, especially IBS (irritable bowel syndrome) or even more serious IBD (irritable bowel disease, Crohn's, Colitis Ulcerosa) or just simply want to have a better health.

The amount of surgery operations are rapidly increasing in the western world. Whatever we are doing or, maybe more specifically what we are exposing ourselves to through our food and the chemicals around us is causing us greater illnesses than we have ever experienced.

Life should be simple, we all want to live healthy and happy lives. To a large extent, you often do not realise how precious health is overall until you lose it. I lost my health and almost my life to Crohn's disease between 2003 and 2004 when I was a little more than 30 years old. With a strong will to live healthy again and through perseverance I made some major changes which paid off. I'm now a much healthier person than I was during my childhood years and up until my 30's, which truly should not be the case. Sickness should not be a part of any child's life.

I want to encourage anyone that has been diagnosed with IBS or IBD that they should keep all options open and they must not forget the power of our own will and the power of our own body's ability to heal. For me my recovery has been a dream come true up until now, although we must remember that this disease can always surprise us in good and bad ways. I hope you can also keep your dreams alive despite the illnesses you may be going through. You are very welcome to join me on this journey as I continue to learn and make choices, make mistakes, enjoy, love and grow as a person.

# THE WORLD NEEDS ROLEMODELS
# WILL YOU
# BE ONE?

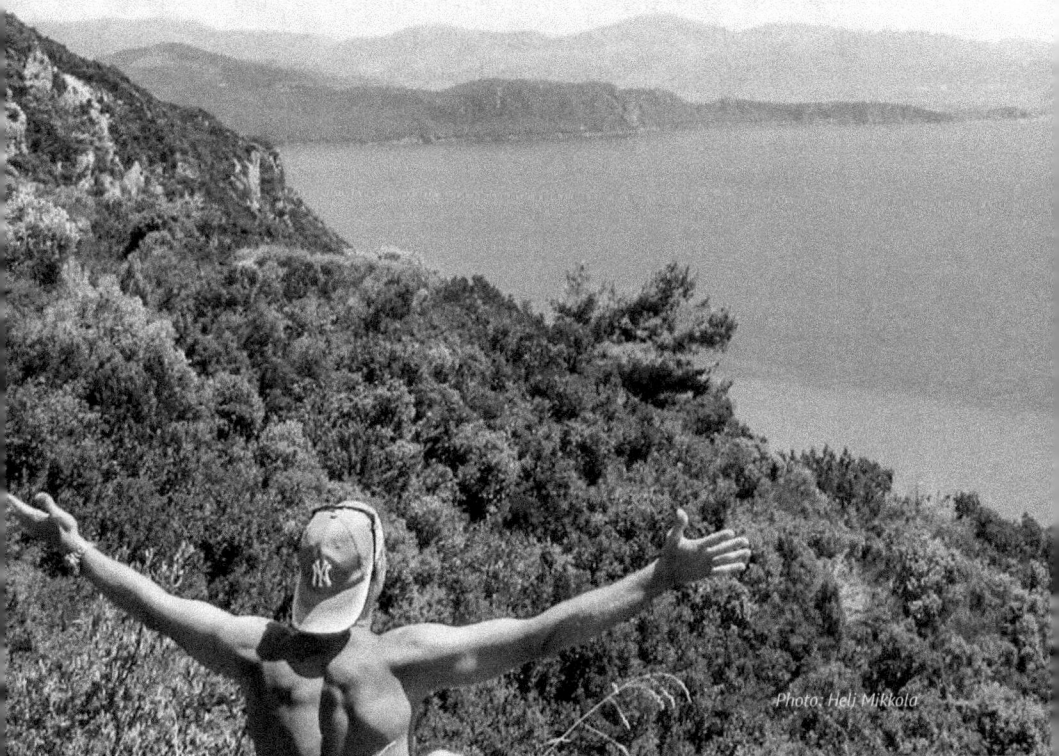

# FOREWORD

I have to admit that I was too naive and lazy to treat my body with respect before I decided to change my life. After having read this book I hope you are motivated to treat yourself with love. Do not wait until the sickness takes over. You need to be in charge of your own body.

If our bowel system is not working well it makes our lives very challenging. One day of having diarrhea doesn't have a great impact on your life but when it continues for weeks or months it can turn into a nightmare that controls your whole life.

What has been life-changing for me was the Head Surgeon's words in hospital in 2004: "You will come back for your next operation within two to three years". At the time, those words motivated me a great deal and made me to make a decision to take a whole new approach for healing.

Today, I have lived almost symptom-free and drug-free for over a decade since 2004. Before then I didn't have sufficient information about the illness or other choices available besides the use of western medicine, which unfortunately didn't work for me. That's why I have been doing a lot of my own research and discovering alternative remedies in order to survive. Since making the right choices and changes in my life, in 2004 at the age of 35, the quality of my life has improved drastically. Knowledge and experience helps enormously. The biggest learning curve has been to get to know my body and learn to listen to what it is saying and what it is teaching me.

> LEARN FROM OTHERS WHO HAVE WALKED THE PATH BEFORE YOU. BUT BE SMART ENOUGH TO KNOW WHEN TO BREAK AWAY TO CUT YOUR OWN PATH.
>
> NARCISO RODRIGUEZ

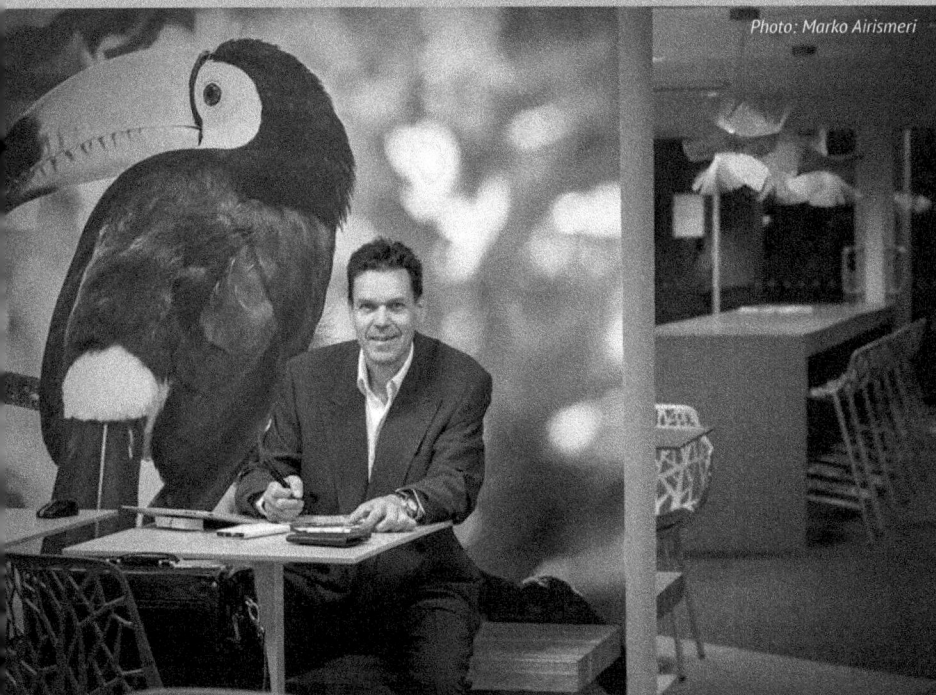

Photo: Marko Airismeri

# BACKGROUND: TOMMI SUNDQVIST

**COUNTRY OF BIRTH:** Turku, Finland

**DATE OF BIRTH:** 1969

**PROFESSION:** Information-Technology-worker, Nutritionist, Sports masseur, entrepreneur and lecturer.

**HOBBIES:** Travelling, being in the nature, aikido, yoga, ice-hockey, gym etc.

**TODAY:** I live a healthy and active life with my loved ones, my wife Heli and our beautiful daughters and our beloved rescued husky-dog. We are also a foster family for children in need.

**CONTACT:** nakedgut@gmail.com

# I AM FOREVER GRATEFUL

For having these warm-hearted individuals helping me with this project.
My beautiful wife Heli who has been beside me throughout the hardest moments. Without you I would not be here writing this story, you mean the world to me. Our children, Mia-Marie and Meri-Helene for supporting and understanding me. My mother Tarja, who has always shown how much she loves and cares. My relatives, Aunt Päivi, my grandmother, my brother Henri, and everybody who has helped me along the way and all my friends, who have shown me much support and understanding.

MY TRANSLATORS:

Liz Barrington, who has done a great job checking the grammar. Eveliina Valkeapää (Master of Arts, French and English teacher, health care secretary) who has done great job earlier with the grammar.

PROOFREADER:

Janette St. Pierre (wholesale distributor of organic health foods and herbal medicine in Eugene Oregon USA). She knows what it means to heal the body through natural and more gentle remedies, without the damaging side effects of synthetic drugs.

PICTURES:

Marko Airismeri (Professional photographer) whose beautiful pictures powerfully convey the message better than I could have ever imagined. Other photos are either from image banks, our family albums or Sanna Kostamo´s library.

LAYOUT:

Sanna Kostamo (photographer and a talented designer), who has been very helpful in this journey. She also shares her great story in this book.

ADDITIONAL THANKS GO TO ALL THE DOCTORS WHO HAVE TREATED ME. THE SPORT TEAMS, HOKUTO AIKIDO, PLAYBOYS ICE-HOCKEY TEAM, SUNKEN LOGS FREEDIVING ETC. MY COLLEAGUES AND NUMEROUS PEOPLE ON INTERNET WHO HAVE INSPIRED ME IN SEARCH OF A BETTER HEALTH.

# WHY I CHOSE MY OWN PATH

For starters: I simply had no other choice than change the course!

I know there are millions of people like me who are searching for relief from stomach and intestine problems like IBS (irritable bowel syndrome) and to more severe conditions such as IBD (Inflammatory bowel disease), Crohn´s disease and Ulcerative Colitis. IBD especially can be very painful and even deadly if not effectively treated.

The main message what I have learned is this: It is possible to heal. What has amazed me even more is that it is possible to live life symptom-free by making different choices. I did not know this important fact 15 years ago.

In this book I discuss the various options that have helped me enormously. I noticed that the help may be there, you just have to find the right one that works for you. I realised that if I wanted to live healthier, I needed to take off the blinkers and think outside the box.

When you read this, you will understand why I had to choose a different way of healing other than relying totally on western medicine. I was totally pro-medicine, I had even studied international marketing of medicine and I got very close to working in a big Pharma company, but destiny created a very different path to what I had originally expected.

Small choices we make every day have a greater meaning in our life than we may ever understand. Sometimes choices are not given; at least it felt like that, but practically I was forced to change my opinion about how I need to heal. I know that I may not get rid of Crohn´s completely, but my main goal is to live a symptom-free life. I had to wait until I was 35 years before I really understood that this is possible.

The decision I made was not an easy one and did not happen overnight. Although in 2004 I was determined about one thing: I would do whatever I could in my power to be healthy again.

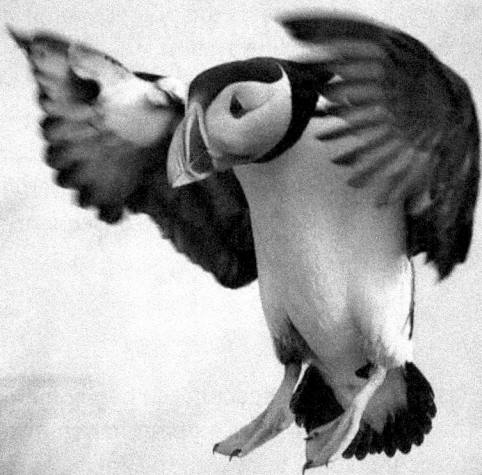

Photo: Marko Airismeri

WHEN THE TIME IS RIGHT
THINGS WILL FALL INTO PLACE

# GUT BACTERIA IS CRUCIAL IN OUR LIFE

I admit, I did not pay any attention to the healthy and balanced bacteria before. Years of neglected behavior, mainly as unhealthy food choices like sugar, gluten etc. were nibbling my gut bacteria until I realised how essential it is to our well-being.

Our gut is a mystery like Amazon, because there is so much that surprises us over and over again. If Amazon is the planet's lungs and natural pharmacy, our gut is the mother of our immune system.

The size of your intestines is huge, if opened it is equivalent to a basketball court. Microbes in the gut weigh between 1–2,7 kg and there are around 100 billion of them. If you destroy the balance with undernourished and processed food, sooner than later you will carry the consequences possibly in different illnesses, autoimmunity diseases etc.

## NATURAL BIRTH

Bacterias have a huge impact in the beginning of our lives. A vaginal birth gives the newborn baby much better immunity than C-section birth and protects the intestinal tract with the bacterias it gets from mother's vaginal and intestinal flora (at least Bifidobacterium, Lactobasillus and Escheria coli). Babies born through natural childbirth are more alert and show more interest in breastfeeding once delivered to the world.

## C-SECTION

Those who are born via C-section/caesarean section loose important bacterias right in the beginning and have lower immunity, so they need lots of healthy bacteria added in their breast milk. Caesarean also increases the levels of skin-associated bacteria including Staphylococcus. The goal is to give a safe birth both to mom and baby, so sometimes C-section is necessary, so do not blame anyone if that option is taken.

## MOTHER´S MILK

Another important thing to our immune system is breast milk and bacterias have a big role in it too. Oligosaccharides that are present in mother's breast milk also promote the growth of two healthy bacterias, Lactobacillus and Bifidobacterium. These bacterias have a big impact to our immune system and to our health and future.

Breast milk is ultimately the best source of nutrition for a new baby. Many components in breast milk help build immunity and protect your precious baby against infection and disease. The proteins in breast milk are more easily digested than in formula or cow's milk. The calcium and iron in breast milk are also more easily absorbed.

# NOT KNOWING HAS FORCED ME TO MAKE DIFFICULT DECISIONS

How much has IBS/IBD affected my life and that of others too? The answer is very much so.

Life is a big teacher, it offers you different paths every single day. The hard part is choosing the "right" paths to follow. Besides, with all the "incorrect" or more challenged paths, what we very often do not seek are those routes that educate us even more so that the end result is often better when you look at it from a different angle and with patience.

I used to be a patient with no patience. It takes patience and perseverance to heal. I did not stop to think what is the real problem until I was almost forced to do so. Stomach pain had been a part of me for my entire childhood and they couldn't find a reason until I was aged 19. The partial cause I was given was related to my genes, because my grandfather also had similar symptoms.

Crohn's disease has strongly influenced me throughout. I have to admit, I was very much against having my own children because of the disease. When I was a young adult, very sick and at the same time I should have been thinking about having children, that scenario was just too much for me. How could a sick person take care of children? Do I want to take the risk of my children having the same sickness? If I had known that I could affect my own Crohn's symptoms so much, I would have made different choices. Anyone who has children knows that these kind of decisions are not made easily. It has been the most difficult choice in my life so far. I have two beautiful daughters from Heli's side and we are a foster family today, so I can live like a loving parent. There are numerous children who need support, so even if I do not have any biological children of my own, there are plenty of children out there in need of love and care. One experienced specialist in child, adolescent and adult psychiatry told me a great wisdom regarding how to raise a child: "The most important gift you can give to the child is a healthy self-esteem."

THE MOST
IMPORTANT GIFT
YOU CAN GIVE TO
THE CHILD IS
A HEALTHY
SELF-ESTEEM.

# DIGESTIVE SYSTEM – IN A NUTSHELL

Digestion is crucial for the body, so in order to understand just the basics, let's take a look at the route food has to go through in your system. Digestion's job is to break down the food gradually into smaller components in order for the body to utilise the nutrients easily.

## 1. MOUTH

### CHEW WELL!

Digestion starts in the mouth. Chewing breaks the food into pieces that are more easily digested, saliva with its enzymes mixes with food to start the process of breaking it down into a form your body can absorb and readily use as efficiently as possible. Binge eating is not good for the digestion, so chew your food well. Our only job is to use enough time for chewing (20–30 times before swallowing the food), the rest of digestion is automatic. Our body is amazing!

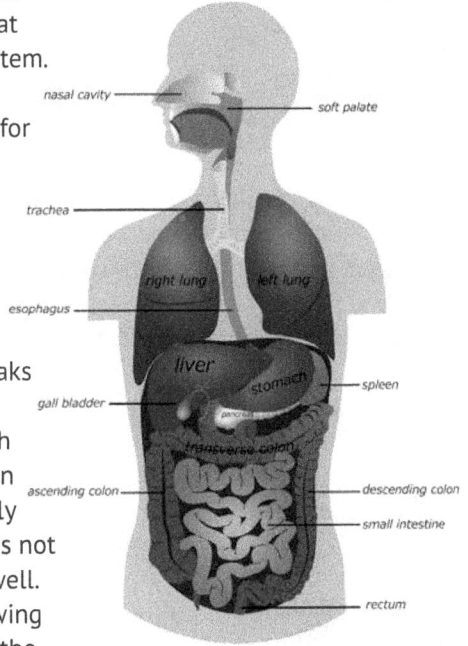

nasal cavity
soft palate
trachea
right lung
left lung
esophagus
liver
stomach
spleen
gall bladder
pancreas
transverse colon
ascending colon
descending colon
small intestine
rectum

## 2. THROAT (PHARYNX)

The throat (pharynx) is a muscular tube that runs from the back of your nose down into your neck. It contains three (3) sections: the nasopharynx, oropharynx and laryngopharynx, which is also called the hypopharynx.

## 3. ESOPHAGUS (FOOD PIPE)

The esophagus is a muscular tube extending from the throat to the stomach. The average length is 10 in / 25 cm, about the length of a long cucumber. It performs a wave of sequenced contractions. Those moves are called peristalsis. It moves the food from the throat to the stomach. When you swallow food, the upper esophageal sphincter (bundle of muscles) opens automatically which prevents the air you breathe going into stomach.

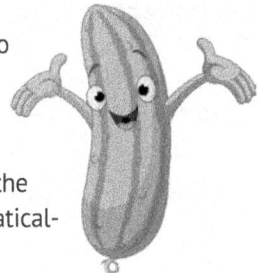

That muscle keeps the food going forward. There is also the lower esophageal sphincter that is the last gateway before the stomach. This ingenious lower "gate" prevents the stomach acids returning to the esophagus.

## 4. STOMACH

| Food transit time in the stomach | 4 to 5 hours |
| --- | --- |

The stomach holds, mixes and grinds the food within its strong muscular walls. The stomach secretes important enzymes and acid, so that the process of breaking down the food can continue. After stomach digestion, the consistency of food is liquid or paste. Adult stomach can hold food and liquid after a meal up to 1 liter to even 4 liters (almost a gallon).

## 5A. SMALL INTESTINE

| Food transit time in the small intestine | 15 min–5 hrs |
| --- | --- |

The small intestine is made up of three segments.

I) The duodenum, which breaks down the food.

II & III) The jejunum and the ileum which are mainly in charge of the absorption of nutrients. The length of the small intestine can be 6 m / 20 ft, which is equivalent to the average length of a green anaconda, one of the longest snakes in the world. The process of breaking down food continues by using enzymes released by the pancreas and bile. In a study the average transit time was 1 hr 24 mins. (AJR - American Journal of Roentgenology).

## 5B. PANCREAS, LIVER AND GALLBLADDER

- The pancreas secretes enzymes that break down protein, fat, and carbohydrates within the food we eat.
- The liver purifies the blood coming from the small intestine and it makes/secretes bile.
- The gallbladder stores bile.

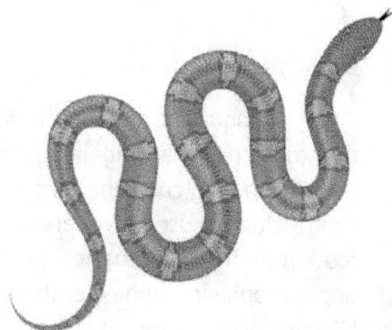

- Bile helps with digestion and eliminates waste products from the blood. They each have an essential role which should not be underestimated.

## 6. LARGE INTESTINE, COLON

| Food transit time in the large intestine | 30–40 hrs |
| --- | --- |

The colon absorbs water and minerals. The colon's microflora/bacteria helps digestion, promotes vital nutrient production, maintains pH (acid-base) balance and prevents the proliferation of harmful bacteria. Gut microbiota is the absolute cornerstone of our health. These healthy organisms can weigh up to 2 kg and include tens of trillions of micro-organisms, which are more than 1000 different species of bacteria with more than 3 million genes (150 times more than human genes). One third of our gut microbiota is common to most people, while two thirds are specific to each one of us, just like our fingerprints are unique. The colon is approximately a 5-feet / 1,55 cm long muscular tube.

The colon connects the cecum (the first part of the large intestine) to the rectum (the last part of the large intestine). It is made up of the cecum, the ascending (right) colon, the transverse (across) colon, the descending (left) colon, and the sigmoid colon (for its "S" shape), which connects to the rectum.
Women usually have a longer colon. A study done by The Department of Endoscopy, St. Mark's Hospital, London, England found out that total colonic length was greater in women (median 5 feet/155 cm) compared to men (median, 4,75 feet/ 145 cm). That may explain why colonoscopy is a more difficult for women than for men.

Stool, or fecal waste left over from the digestive process, is passed through the colon by means of peristalsis (contractions), first in a liquid state and ultimately in solid form as the water is removed from the stool. A stool is stored in the sigmoid colon until a 'mass movement' empties it into the rectum once or twice a day. It normally takes about 36 hours for stool to get through the colon. The stool itself is mostly food debris and bacteria. These bacterias perform several useful functions, such as synthesizing various vitamins, processing waste products and food particles, and protecting against harmful microorganisms.

## 7. RECTUM

When the descending colon becomes full of stool or feces, it empties its contents into the rectum to begin the process of elimination. Although the rectum is a small organ, it is a very important one with a critical function. Imagine if the rectum was not working, your life would become miserable very quickly.

## DIFFERENCES BETWEEN HUMAN AND CARNIVORE

- Human intestine: 9 times of the body length and weak hydrochloric acid
- Carnivore intestine: Up to 3 times the body length and strong hydrochloric acid
- Based on our teeth and intestines, humans are designed to eat mostly FRUITS, VEGETABLES AND NUTS and carnivores MEAT.

### HOW THE COLON SHOULD IDEALLY WORK

A person with a healthy colon will have 2 to 3 bowel movements per day, shortly after each meal taken. Elimination should be complete and easy. The stool should be light brown in color, long and large diameter. There should be no offensive odor and it should break apart with toilet flushing.

This describes the normal function of a healthy colon, it perhaps sounds like a fairytale. In this society, how many of us can really say "my gut works perfectly all the time"?

What is your own personal food transit time? One way to find out is to eat beetroot – it will show you the speed of your metabolism literally from top to bottom.

# IBS – IRRITABLE BOWEL SYNDROME

| | |
|---|---|
| WHAT IS IT? | It is when the muscles in your large intestine contract faster or slower than normal causing uncomfortable symptoms. |
| SYMPTOMS? | Pain, cramping, trapped wind, sudden bouts of diarrhea and constipation etc. |
| PREVALENCE | 10–23 % of population worldwide have IBS |
| CONDITION | Chronic. No inflammation, bleeding or cancer |

It is estimated that even 23% of worldwide population have IBS, a digestive system disorder. IBS occurs when muscles in your large intestine contract faster or slower than normal. This causes pain, cramping, trapped wind, sudden bouts of diarrhea and constipation. It is a very uncomfortable syndrome that has a great impact on our everyday life.

Most of the people who have mild symptoms of IBS never go to see a doctor, or else they may postpone having it checked out for as long as possible, so the amount of people that we know have been diagnosed with suffering from IBS may just be the tip of the iceberg. The cost to society is huge. Direct medical expenses and indirect costs associated with loss of productivity and work absenteeism is estimated to be at least $21 billion annually.

If loose stools are the main symptoms of your IBS, a few changes to your diet may help. Avoid these for two weeks: Chocolate, alcohol, caffeine, carbonated drinks, sorbitol (found in sugarless gum and mints) and excessive fructose (around 50% of table sugar and high-fructose corn syrup).

Doctors may suggest you to take a Cal-protectin test and a colonoscopy to help rule out other conditions such as Crohn's disease, ulcerative colitis etc.

You can take a simple stool test in a laboratory to check your Cal-protectin levels. Faecal Calprotectin is a biomarker and screens out patients with IBS who do not require endoscopies. The levels of fecal calprotectin can be used to evaluate the response to a specific treatment, to screen asymptomatic patients, and to predict inflammatory bowel disease relapses.

Calprotectin levels can predict clinical relapse with a 90% sensitivity and 83% accuracy. Results that show above 50 mg/kg will require a re- test and over 100 mg/kg may indicate colorectal inflammation. More about my personal Cal-pro experience in "My story"-section.

# IBD – INFLAMMATORY BOWEL DISEASE

| | |
|---|---|
| WHAT IS IBD? | Diagnoses as Crohn's and Ulcerative colitis. Involves chronic inflammation of all or part of your digestive tract. |
| SYMPTOMS? | Pain, cramping, trapped wind, gassiness, sudden bouts of diarrhea and constipation etc. |
| PREVALENCE | A global disease with increasing prevalence, minimum of 5 M patients worldwide |
| CONDITION | Chronic with inflammation, bleeding or possibly cancer |

Inflammatory bowel disease or IBD has spread worldwide, predominately across Northern-America, Europe and Australia. At least five million people live with Crohn's disease and ulcerative colitis – all conditions known as inflammatory bowel diseases (IBD). Main symptoms include: low abdominal pain, diarrhea and even bloody diarrhea, weight loss, anemia, loose stools, sudden bowel urges, bloating, gas.

IBD is more severe than IBS. IBD is a chronic disease with inflammation, irritation and bloody diarrhea. It can cause bloody lacerations within any part of the Gastrointestinal tract, from mouth to anus. It can be fatal if not well-treated. IBD is the same as:

• Crohn's disease (usually in small intestine)
• Ulcerative colitis (usually in large intestine)
• Indeterminate colitis (when it's difficult to distinguish between Crohn and Colitis)

Most people with IBS will never develop IBD. Still, it may be tricky because a person who has been diagnosed with IBD may display IBS-like symptoms. Both

IBS and IBD are considered chronic (ongoing) conditions. Crohn and Colitis patients both have an inflammation, whereas IBS does not cause inflammation.

Crohn's disease and ulcerative colitis are different types of IBD. The symptoms of these two illnesses are quite similar, but the areas affected in the gastrointestinal tract (GI tract) are different. Crohn's most commonly affects the end of the small bowel (the ileum) and the beginning of the colon, but it may affect any part of the gastrointestinal (GI) tract, from mouth to anus. Ulcerative colitis is limited to the colon, otherwise known as the large intestine. If you have any of these symptoms, contact a doctor to find out what the problem is.

About 45% of people with ulcerative colitis and up to 75% of people with Crohn's disease will eventually require surgery. Some people with these conditions have the option to choose surgery, while for others, surgery is an absolute necessity due to complications and seriousness of their disease.

Crohn and Colitis are treated with medication and surgery, although in a survey in Germany over 50% of patients reported that they had used or presently use CAM (complementary and alternative medicine) to help treat their condition. Among IBS sufferers, 40% reported not to be satisfied with the drugs and remedies they currently use to treat their IBS symptoms. So there is a significant amount of people seeking other solutions to ease their symptoms.

It is a disease that has spread all over the western world. To increase awareness of this condition, there is plenty of IBD-info within the market, such as "World IBD Day" that is held on 19th May each year. World IBD Day is led by patient organisations representing at least 35 countries across four continents including Argentina, Australia, Brazil, Canada, EU nations (including the umbrella organisation EFCCA), Israel, Japan, New Zealand, the United States of America and more.

# LEAKY GUT
# – THE LINK TO ALL AUTOIMMUNE DISEASES?

| | |
|---|---|
| WHAT IS IT? | It is when the cell lining mainly in the small intestine, becomes "leaky" due to an inflammation. |
| SYMPTOMS? | Pain, cramping, trapped wind, sudden bouts of diarrhea and constipation etc. |
| PREVALENCE | Unknown. Intestinal permeability is a factor in many diseases, such as Crohn's, ulcerative colitis, multiple sclerosis, fibromyalgia, chronic fatique, celiac disease, Type 1&2 diabetes, rheumatoid arthritis etc. |
| CONDITION | Chronic |

"Leaky gut" syndrome is a very common disorder in which the cells lining the intestines become "leaky" due to inflammation. The lining is normally tightly-sealed. However when the gut becomes leaky, this is due to the abnormally large spaces present between the cells of the gut wall that allow toxic material like parasites and other harmful invaders into the bloodstream that would normally be eliminated. Leaky gut may even play a role in neurodegenerative diseases like Parkinson's. Changes in intestinal tight junction permeability are associated with industrial food additives (neurotoxins, GMO, antibiotics, rx-drugs) which may explain the rising incidence of autoimmune diseases. One way to test for a leaky gut is a zonulin test. High levels of zonulin can enlarge the openings in the intestinal wall. A food allergy test is also helpful. Larazotide acetate (INN-202) is a new (on trials 2018) promising drug for tightening the intercellular junctions.

There are many threats to our gut:

> Stress, alcohol, tobacco, misuse of drugs, overuse of non-steroidal drugs (ibuprofen etc.), H2 blockers, chemotherapy, vaccines, processed foods (additives, hydrogenated oils etc.), allergies, infections and parasites. Gmo, pesticides, chemicals, Reduced stomach acid, yeast overgrowth, imbalance of bacteria, bad mouth hygiene. Environmental threats, mold etc. etc.

Overuse of these problematic substances can damage the seal between cells and make the gut leak harmful substances into the bloodstream.

Excerpts below are from Carrageenan - New Studies Reinforce Link to Inflammation, Cancer and Diabetes. Updated report by The Cornucopia Institute / April 2016.

Some food additives are very problematic to our health. Three examples include:
1. Carrageenan (also called Irish Moss)
2. Polysorbate 80
3. Carboxymethylcellulose

Health problems linked to them: Cancer, GI inflammation, malignant tumors, diabetes, colitis and metabolic syndrome. Eating emulsifiers on a daily basis may promote chronic, low-level inflammation. Cut most of the emulsifiers out of your food today! Since inflammation is at the root of most diseases, this is a major finding.

## A LITTLE MORE ABOUT CARRAGEENAN

It is extracted from red seaweed and used in our foods, medicine, toothpaste and even alcohol as a binder, thickening agent and stabilizer. It adds zero nutritional value or flavor, it has a controversial reputation as an additive that damages the digestive system. The National Organics Standards Board voted already in November 2016 to remove carrageenan from the list of substances allowed in organic food. The United States Department of Agriculture (USDA) has the final say in November 2018, Food Safety News informs.

I remember once at the supermarket when a lady brought back the organic apple juice to the counter. She thought the product was spoiled because it was a cloudy juice with bits and pieces on the bottom. In this case both the staff and customers need guidance too. Simple "Shake well before the consumption"-label could be enough and carrageenan is not needed.

Carrageenan affects the body to trigger an immune reaction, which leads to inflammation in the gastrointestinal system. The amazing thing is that scientists have been warning about the use of carrageenan from the sixties, over four decades. Studies have repeatedly shown that food-grade carrageenan causes gastrointestinal inflammation, intestinal lesions and even malignant tumors. Almost 4000 research pages show that it is inducing inflammation, so it is quite shocking why you find it in so many products in the supermarket.

## LIST OF THE FOODS THAT OFTEN HAVE CARRAGEENAN:

- Dairy (ice-cream, whipped cream, even squeezable yogurt for children!)
- Dairy alternatives that are supposed to be healthy (almond-, hemp-, coconutmilk)
- Meats (sliced turkey)
- Nutritional drinks (Slimfast etc.)
- Prepared foods (microwaveable foods, frozen pizzas)
- Vitamins (chewable)
- Canned pet food

Eliminate carrageenan from your diet and you may end these symptoms: The painful stomach cramps, multiple body aches, awful bloating symptoms, spastic colon, IBS and even ulcerative colitis may be stopped.

Please note that when you go for X-Ray and drink the barium drink, it may contain carrageenan too.

If we know all these details, why are we willingly adding this and other controversial substances into our foods?

# 5 DIAGNOSES TO CHECK

When you have gut problems, these 5 diagnoses are good to check to rule each one out:

1. Lactose-intolerance
2. Fructose allergy
3. Dysbiosis. Imbalance in the intestines, especially if you have taken lots of antibiotics in the past. (Stool test: Genova Diagnostics – GI effect)
4. Overproduction of yeast. Substances that kill yeast: Garlic, oregano, pau d'arco, berberin (source: Oregon Grape Root).
5. SIBO (small intestinal bacteria overgrowth)

If you have constipation, low stomach acidity or simply too much stress could be the cause. SIBO normally occurs in the large intestine, but it can be found in the small intestine too.

SIBO, is defined as an increase in the quantity of bacteria, and/or changes in the types of bacteria present in the small bowel. Patients who are immunodeficient, whether due to an abnormal antibody response or T-cell response, are prone to bacterial overgrowth, so it is very common to have SIBO if you have IBS or IBD. Studies suggest that as much as 80% of gut patients can have SIBO.

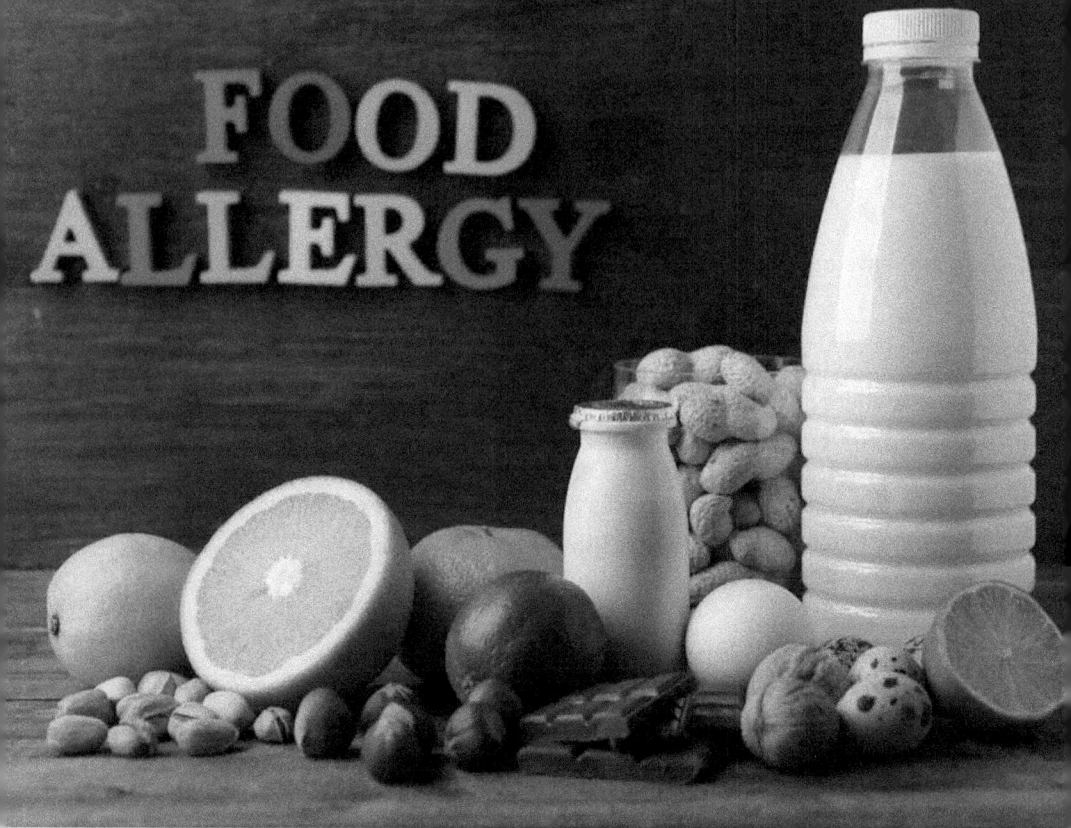

# FOOD ALLERGY

"FOOD ALLERGIES AMONG CHILDREN HAVE INCREASED BY APPROXIMATELY 50% IN JUST 14 YEARS (1997-2011)."

# AUTOIMMUNE DISEASES ARE SOARING

"Food allergies among children have increased by approximately 50% in just 14 years (1997–2011), according to a study released in 2013 by the US Centers for Disease Control and Prevention."

"Children Diagnosed with an Autoimmune Condition or Celiac Disease have a 40% increased risk of committing suicide compared to a non-celiac child." (betrayalseries.com)

"This is the first generation of Americans that is expected to have a shorter lifespan than their parents. Autoimmune disease is why the IQ of children is going down while developmental disorders are going up. This is why one in two people are getting cancer and 25% of people are losing their minds to dementia." (wholebodyhealth.org)

These are serious topics. So, what is happening in our world? Why is our body suddenly attacking our own immune system and why are these diseases affecting our minds so strongly too? What has changed so drastically in just a few decades?

The fact is that if our gut is bombarded with substances that are not natural to our own body, this affects our minds too in a long run. In the last fifty years our connection to nature has changed. We are living further away from it and forgetting that we should live with nature, not against it. Today we are living in a world that is full of chemicals. There have been many changes to our food and water during the past few decades: we are consuming large quantities of preservatives, flavors, colorings, food additives, hormones, antibiotics and growth hormones that are being used in food production. Today, more than 30,000 chemicals are now marketed in the European Union alone. Eventually they will get inside us through the air, soil and water, no matter how we try to protect ourselves.

Food and drink alone contain around 1,000 different chemicals and not all are good for you. The toxic chemicals are present in nearly every home, packed into couches, chairs, clothing, cleaning products, cosmetics, toys etc. They are everywhere. Some chemicals are meant to protect us from bigger disasters, like flame retardants, however we are being exposed to high levels of these toxic chemicals every single day. To prevent a terrible accident you need to be exposed to yet another toxic threat. Sometimes it's tough to choose what is right and wrong. What's more, climate changes with rising temperatures make smog pollution even worse.

All chemicals combine a major threat to our immune system. As Michael Conrad from the Hill Street Blues TV-series had said in 1990's: "Let's be careful out there!".

## HELP STRENGTHEN YOUR IMMUNE SYSTEM

What you can do to protect and strengthen your immune system is eat organic food and lots of antioxidant-rich ie. vitamin-rich food that protects you from harmful free radical damage. Great sources of antioxidants are fruit, berries, vegetables and superfoods. Also most spices are high in ORAC-values (a health value of a food / antioxidant value).

## WHAT HAPPENS DURING AN AUTOIMMUNE ATTACK?

The blood cells in the body's immune system help protect against harmful substances. When your autoimmune system is getting mixed signals, it does not recognize the difference between healthy tissue and antigens. An antigen is any substance that causes your immune system to produce antibodies against it. Then the body starts to attack its own tissues when trying to destroy them.

An antigen may be any foreign material from the environment, such as chemicals, bacteria, viruses or pollen. An antigen may also be formed inside the body. An autoimmune disorder may also result in the abnormal growth of an organ or changes in organ function.

Autoimmune diseases are spreading fast and are a major health problem around the world. The numbers may surprise you but, for instance in America, autoimmune diseases affect up to 50 million Americans, according to the American Autoimmune Related Diseases Association (AARDA). In comparison, heart diseases affect 22 million and cancer up to 9 million Americans.

## PHARMACEUTICAL COMPANIES ARE ALSO INTERESTED IN THE GROWING NUMBERS

The fact is that there is huge business in this field too. As our western lifestyle spreads all around the world, so do autoimmune diseases. The increasing prevalence of autoimmune diseases can be seen in the global autoimmune disease diagnostics markets too. North America dominates the global autoimmune disease diagnostics market, followed by Europe. China and India are expected to have the fastest growing markets in the next five years. South American countries such as Brazil and Mexico are the regions that have significant potential for growth due to developing medical infrastructure, high disposable income and rising prevalence of autoimmune diseases.

Some of the major companies operating in autoimmune disease diagnostic market are Abbott Laboratories Ltd, Active Biotech, AstraZeneca plc, Amgen, Inc., Eli Lilly and Company, 4SC AG, Bristol-Myers Squibb Company, Pfizer, Inc., GlaxoSmithKline plc, F. Hoffmann-La Roche Ltd., and Johnson & Johnson Ltd.

## SCIENCE IS HELPING US TO LIVE HEALTHIER

> SCIENCE IS AT ITS BEST A GREAT TOOL TO HELP US BECOME HEALTHIER. BUT WE STILL NEED TO TAKE RESPONSIBILITY FOR LIVING HEALTHIER EVERY DAY, BY MAKING BETTER CHOICES.

Sometime very soon if it's not happening already technology will find answers as to how to avoid getting sicknesses and also how to live longer. Google-backed Calico is searching for genetic trends of human longevity. Collaboration with AncestryDNA can provide access to a unique combination of resources that will enable Calico to develop potentially groundbreaking therapeutic solutions. The extensive research period will identify common patterns in longevity and human heredity through genealogy data.

So just wait and you might see new technology giving us an application or a pill designed personally for you which makes you healthier. What is going to be innovative is when we find ways of preventing detectable diseases well ahead of time.

Immunotherapy / biologic therapy is very interesting too, a cancer treatment that boosts the body's natural defenses to fight the cancer and maybe other chronic inflammatory diseases too. Trials are already happening. QBECO SSI, made from components of inactivated Enteropathic E. coli, aims to restore normal innate immune function in the gastrointestinal track and colon. More info: qubiologics.com

CRISPR/Cas9 and targeted Genome editing is another example. It shows us a new era in molecular biology. It is a method where you can modify genomes.

Genome editing is being studied for cancer treatment and blood disease, but its usefulness for specific genome recruitment can be endless. If it can help us to live healthier and access is given to everyone, then it would be great. We shall see in the near future who will actually benefit from it.

We have the technology to screen the body and even provide walk-in labs to importantly discover which vitamin and nutritional deficiencies we have but these labs are in limited use. People who have the money can get access to these, but the majority of people can't afford to test themselves. This is where our governments should step in and make it possible.

# SHARING
# IS CARING

2004–2005 I found real hope for making a full recovery
from one specific book: Jordan S. Rubin´s "Patient Heal
Thyself": This is a Remarkable Health Program
that combines Ancient Wisdom with
Ground-breaking Clinical Research

For the first time, someone has now said that it is
possible to heal. When you see and actually understand
there is hope, this is more powerful than anything.  His
book was the first eye-opener for me.

Thank you Mr. Rubin!

After reading the book, I was more convinced than ever
that I have a chance to live a healthier life. Now it is my
turn to give back. Although we can all offer something
unique, you may learn something from my path.

Do not wait like I did. Take every action possible before
the sickness really gets you. Surgery is a huge decision
and should always be the last option, so if possible, read
this before the surgery. Find your own remedy to ease
the symptoms. There is hope.

Stressful situations in our lives affect gut bacteria and this may trigger different chronic inflammation diseases. Bacteria also have a memory so having a simple fecal test can help us to diagnose diseases. .

If I think about the stressful and painful situations from my childhood, there are two painful events that stick out. I was four years when I had to see the divorce that my parents went through. Another one was when I was bullied and beaten at school at the age of seven. Those incidents have left a mark in my memory and in the gut too.

From the age of eight I had a more stable childhood living with my mom and my brother. I often saw my dad and spent a lot of time with my grandparents especially in their summer cottage in Kemiö. My best memories are from the time we spent in our summer homes in Kemiö and Nauvo. Although they are in different locations, they are both located in the Western Finland province. They are both beautiful and on top of that Nauvo has 3000 smaller islands and rocky reefs in a very unique archipelago, which is where we always take our guests that come from abroad.

During my childhood and up until 1987 when I was 18, I suffered with IBS and inexplicable symptoms. I understand and know today that eating lots of sugary sweets and processed foods had a major impact on my health, making me sick. I was eating loads of unhealthy carbohydrates (sweets) that had very little nutrition. Eating candy was a lot of fun for me when I was a kid, but I also had to pay a huge price for it. Many things in my diet were totally wrong. I was a sugarholic at every level.

Even today, I somehow feel I am not alone; we have been taught for decades to eat sugar, bread, cereal, low fat milk etc. All that a growing child does not need to stay healthy.

Thank God, today the importance of good nutrition is understood better and the wheels of change are turning slowly towards healthier options.
In 1989, at the age of 20, I had every choice available in my life when I lived in Connecticut, USA. I had the time of my life, which meant also I ate in lots of fast food restaurants. McDonald's, Burger King, Taco Bell, Domino's Pizza, Dunkin' Donuts were all my favorites at that time. But suddenly my stomach cramps got more severe in that same year. That was when I got my first bloody diarrhea.
It was a shock of course. So, after about a year, when I returned to Finland for

compulsory military service, I went to the hospital and got a medical diagnosis too; the doctor called it "Ulcerative Colitis", a chronic infection in the large intestine. It was hard for me to accept that diagnosis because it meant I was chronically sick.

I must admit, the diagnosis was at the same time both a relief and a disappointment. The doctor said I was seriously ill and needed hospital-treatment and medication for the rest of my life. Seriously, it was very hard to admit it. When I tried to attend the refresher training after my army service, I found out that my army status had been changed from the normal class-A into class-B. Damn! All I wanted was just to be a normal guy, who enjoys sports like my friends and to be able to do the same things. I was exempted from army service during peace time. It was very frustrating. Mentally I was not ready for class-B. In my 20's I had a denial phase about the sickness lasting for several years.

Later the diagnosis was changed to 'Crohn's Disease', where inflammation is mainly in the small intestine, but the doctor said it could lurk anywhere between mouth and anus. It sounded f**ing great! It was for sure NOT the news I had wanted to hear when I had just turned into adulthood. But the good news was that IBD had actually started my real learning and healing path which has since given me more wisdom and understanding in life.

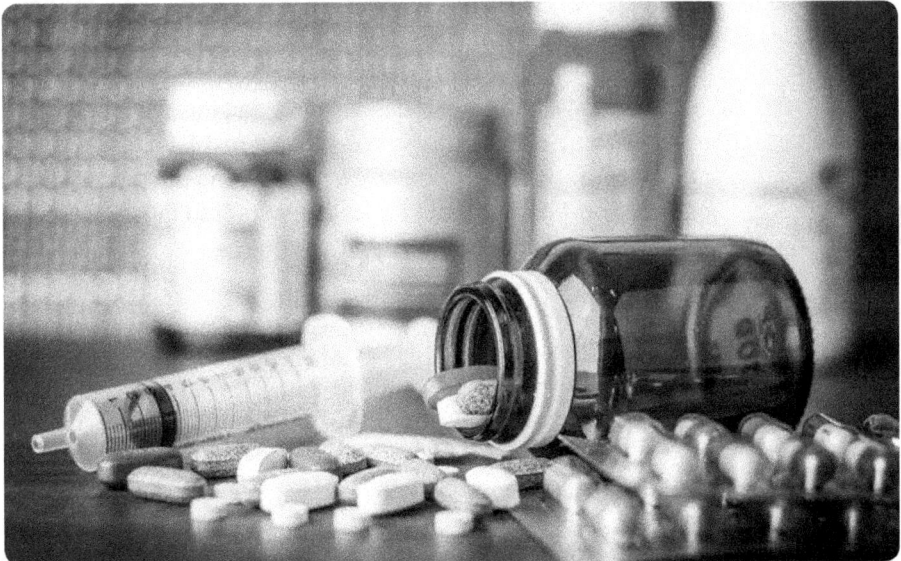

# DOCTOR´S ADVICE

Numerous times I asked the doctors who had treated me, what I could do myself to cure this disease, if there was anything else I could do besides take the medications, go on a special diet perhaps? The answer was always: "You can treat IBD with medicine and then surgery if it gets really bad. Food doesn't play any role in this disease."

Now when I look back at all the doctor's appointments that I had between 1990–2003 I felt that my doctor was truly sorry, because he did not know any other way than to prescribe medicine. Perhaps he did really know deep down that the medicine was not the way to cure this illness? At least not the ones on the market at that time. So, as a doctor who works in a hospital, what should he do? Follow the official guidelines, or risk his job and reputation by giving alternative advice? We never got close at all to getting any alternative advice, he kept the curtain well closed and perhaps it was to protect himself. I am sure he has seen too many cases where patients suffered when there was no cure available. The system does not allow doctors to get to know patients when he has only a few minutes to spare with each case. When hard decisions are made by the doctor, it is also better if the doctor is not too familiar with the patient. Pretty soon I found out this simple law of medicinal health:

*"The fact is that I am the one who is responsible for my overall health and so I am the one who also carries all the consequences, not my doctor. Therefore I am the one who needs to be in charge when any decisions are made."*

From 1990 until 2003, I followed official guidelines by taking medicine and what was the result? Surgery of course. But I was so damn naive that I did not even think you could actually get seriously injured or even die during the surgery, or have complications later. Had I been a fool to trust the system so much? I totally put my health into my doctor´s hands and trusted this was the way I would get better.

Hold on; why did I do that? Is it what we are expected to do? Trust the system blindly? I realized one thing. I have the biggest role in my health, I need to take responsibility and especially I myself have to take back control of my own health, after all it is my body. In the long run, this way I am actually doing a favor to society by making sure I am healthy again, right?

By the time I was 35 years I had been taking loads of medicines, such as Asacol, Prednison, Pentasa, biological medicines etc. without getting any better. At the same time I used to eat unhealthy food just like so many young people do. Little did I know about the consequences. We know that putting low quality oil into our cars will badly affect the engines sooner rather than later. So why on earth would bad quality food not have any effect on our body?

Unhealthy food acts like a poison by flattening intestinal villi and causing infection. When a villus malfunctions, the nutrients do not get absorbed and this bad cycle means that our body becomes very unhealthy. Disease eats into you from the inside out.

Without getting real answers, I decided to start my own research about how to get better from this life threatening disease.

# 3 WAKE-UP CALLS

These 3 chapters include details of the turning points that helped change my lifestyle.

## 1. OSTEOPENIA

In the 1990's, I used to take cortisone to help with my infections, but unfortunately they helped me very little. Corticosteroids are anti-inflammatories, meaning that they decrease levels of inflammation in the body.

That sounds good, but they do have some serious and undesirable side effects which can occur if they are taken for a sustained period of time. After a few years of controlled periods of taking cortisone I was diagnosed with osteopenia. When the doctor said that the use of cortisone had caused the osteopenia, I was stunned! I really did not want my bones to become so weak! It is a condition in which bone mineral density is lower than normal which acts as a precursor to osteoporosis, which is a more serious disease. Osteoporosis occurs when the regeneration of new bone doesn't keep up with the removal of old bone tissue.

Once I got the diagnosis of osteopenia, I stopped using cortisone immediately and the doctor also agreed to that. The precursor was like an alarm clock for me to act. I studied how to promote healthy bones and made sure my diet included enough calcium, multivitamin with vitamin D and K2, magnesium and potassium. I was happy with the results and the decision I had made. The great news was that there was no sign of osteopenia in the following test that was carried out one year later.

You may wonder, can you reverse osteoporosis? Felicia Cosman, MD, Clinical Director of the National Osteoporosis Foundation (NOF) says "Not exactly. But you may be able to curb it. Realistically, we are not talking about complete reversal". So if you do get osteopenia, try to reverse it whilst it is still possible!

## 2. MEDICATION JUST DID NOT WORK FOR ME

In the 1990's I had also been taking loads of medicine called Pentasa over a long period of time with no significant help. Pentasa (mesalamine) affects a substance in the body that causes inflammation, tissue damage and diarrhea to treat active ulcerative colitis.

One of my gastroenterologists told me that the drug I was taking was not helping me with my Colitis, according to studies. What? What did he mean? So, why was I taking it then? That made me very curious. Later I found one review that said: "There was no evidence to suggest that 5-ASA preparations are superior to a placebo for patients with Crohn's disease."

As of 2017, there is no medicine available that suits me without having any obvious side effects, so I am forced to treat myself with alternative unconventional methods.

There is interesting information about the alliance between the medical and science world: "Sometimes we (FDA regulators) have to use experiments that have been carried out in the academic world, perhaps a drug for a rare disease. We simply encounter horrendous problems all the time. When potential drugs enter into the more rigorous pharmaceutical testing processes, 9 out of 10 fail."

Janet Woodcock, a senior official at the Food and Drug Administration (FDA) states in Richard F. Harris book Rigor Mortis: How Sloppy Science Creates Worthless Cures, Crushes Hope, and Wastes Billions.

There are about 7000 known diseases and only about 500 have treatments, many offering just marginal benefits. So there are many challenges when we want to cure ourselves with the help of medicine.

The good news for patients is that other, much gentler therapies are now being taken more seriously. Integrative medicine is the new buzzword in health care. Integrative health and alternative/holistic medicine offer great remedies for optimal health and healing.

Yale University understands the pressure of what students go through with their studies. The Yale Stress Center also offers a variety of stress and wellness programs along with training for individuals and organizations including mindfulness-based stress reduction courses. I am sure it also reaps its returns financially and graduate scores are using these techniques. Yale University was ranked number 8 in the World's Top 10 most prestigious universities in 2016.

Famous hospitals are now offering alternative treatments.
Here are few examples:
1. Cleveland Clinic – Chinese herbal therapy, homeopathy, hypnotherapy, reiki etc.
2. Mayo Clinic – Chinese herbal therapy, meditation, acupuncture, reiki etc.
3. Johns Hopkins – Massage, hypnotherapy, meditation, reiki etc.
4. University of North Carolina – Meditation, art therapy, acupuncture
5. Yale – Chinese herbal therapy, massage, aromatherapy, reiki etc.
The complete list can be found on statnews.com website.

NEW MEDICINES AND HOPE FOR CROHN´S

One of the new treatments available for Crohn's Disease is Mongersen. Giuliani, an Italian pharmaceutical company, conducted a phase 2 clinical study of more than 150 adult patients with Crohn's disease and found that a significant number (even 65%) experienced remission of their inflammatory bowel disease after only 28 days of taking Mongersen. So far, the best results have been with those taking 160 mg daily doses. 10% of patients receiving a placebo treatment experienced remission. Mongersen is a pill unlike other biological medicines like Humira and Remicade which are injections.

## 3. SURGERY – A BLESSING IN DISGUISE

A stormy episode in my life started. Sometimes the tough experiences can and will actually change your life. I now understand that all of this had a bigger meaning in my life. Crohn's disease has been a blessing to me in the long run, although it would seem otherwise. I had to go through hell by constant pain, bloody diarrhea, anemia, blocked bowels, osteopenia, surgery, stoma, peritonitis, MRSA etc. The large quantities of medicines that I was taking were not the solution either. To be honest, I felt lost until the age of 35. I remember one Christmas in particular, in 2003, whilst everyone else in my family were eating Christmas dinner at the table. I was lying on the sofa in agony trying to sip small amounts of blueberry drink and then vomiting, holding my legs up because I was in so much pain. Everything seemed to be getting much worse throughout 2003, so much so that I could hardly eat anything without vomiting. The medicine treatment had failed, so the next in line was surgery.

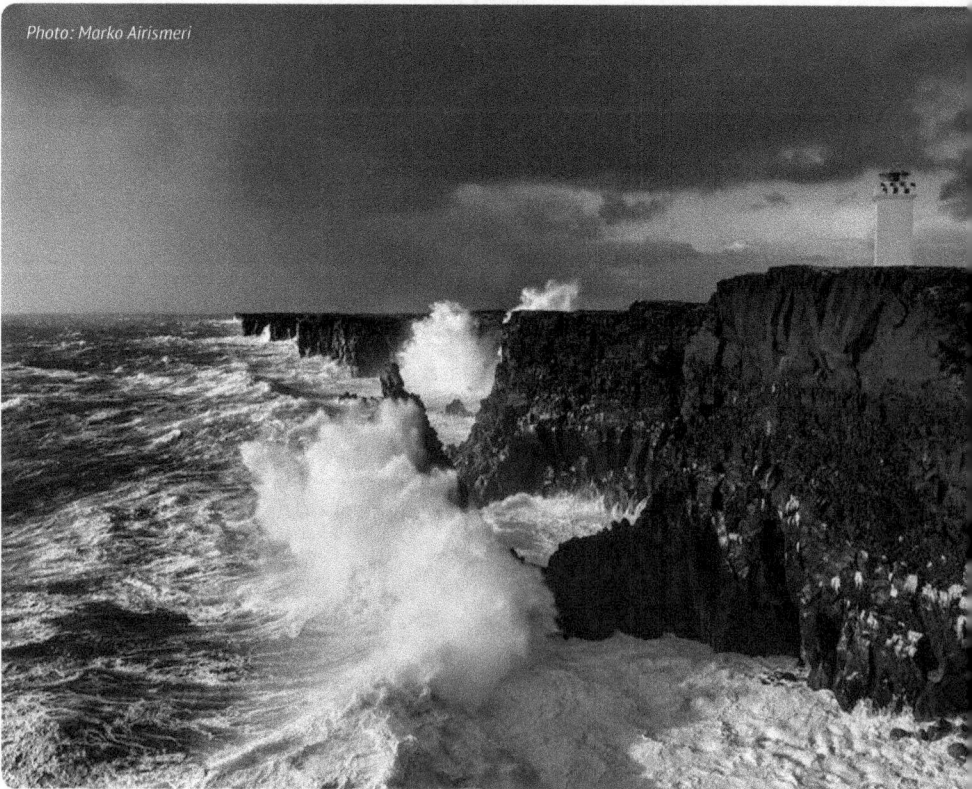

Photo: Marko Airismeri

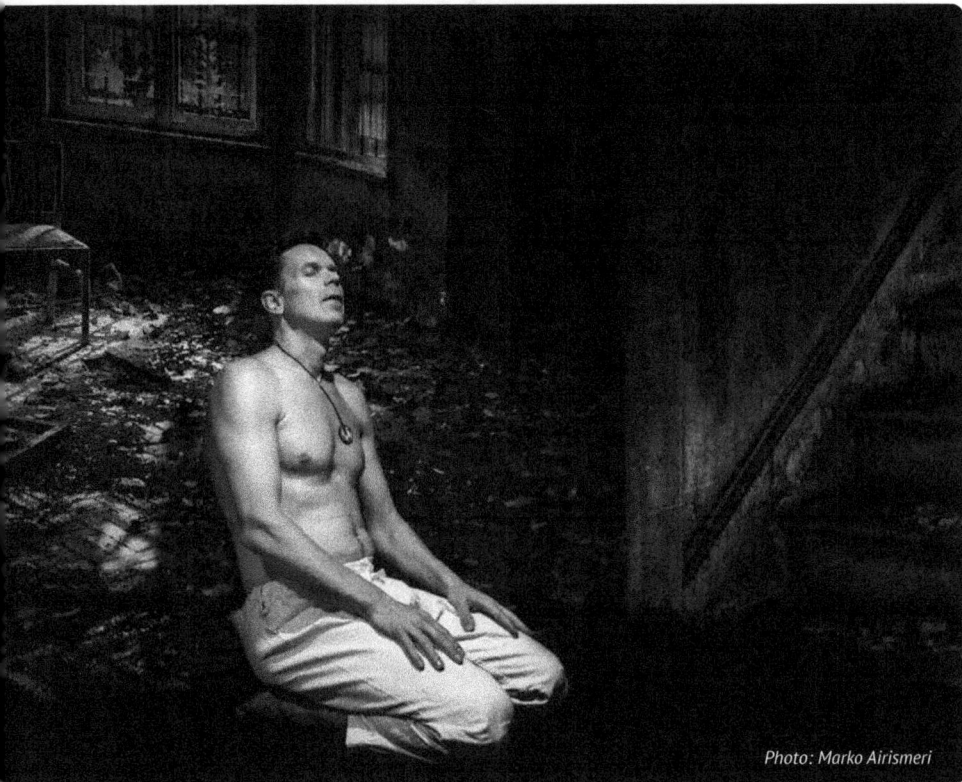

Photo: Marko Airismeri

## 2 MAJOR SURGERIES IN 7 DAYS

On January 5th 2004 the first operation was carried out by two gastrointestinal surgeons (team 1) from Turku University hospital. They made a cut in my mid-belly and the diseased part of my small intestine was removed, which was approximately 47" / 120 cm long. Everything seemed fine on the first day. Later that week I was filled with so much pain (and misery) despite using a pain pump. I thought the pain was meant to disappear out of the picture after the operation. Soon we started to rethink why my belly was turning into a freaking basketball? And for sure, I was not having a baby! Much humour was needed!

Heli tried to hurry up the doctors to examine it closer and to get a simple bloodtest, so that we could see the status of the infection. The answer they gave us was repeated, day after day: "You are not doctors, so do not interfere". Well, it is my body, I have a right to interfere if something is seriously wrong! After a week and after many frustrating promises, when we finally got the bloodtest done and we found out the results the C-reactive protein (CRP) blood test marker (that confirms the presence of inflammation in the body) was alarming (almost 300), and so I was rushed into an emergency operation. Nurses practically flew me into surgery. This time it was clear my life was at stake.

## LUCKY AND BLESSED

I must say I was very fortunate, because just a few hours before the critical CRP results, I was given a permission to go home. But I told the doctor: "I am so sick, I can not even get up from the bed, so how can I go home and survive on my own?" Heli insisted on having more bloodtests done for me. The doctor gave me permission to stay until the CRP levels were checked. Oh boy, if I had gone home in that condition!...I often think how small details can change everything. It felt so lucky and blessed because it felt like angels were with me all the time. The whole thing did not make any sense, why did I survive although there were so many human chances of failing?

11% of those having emergency bowel surgery die within 30 days, according to an audit of the treatment received by 21,000 patients at 192 hospitals in England and Wales.

So, on 12th january 2004 a re-laparotomy was done ie. my belly was opened again by GI-surgeons (team 2). This operation saved my life, thank you surgeons! A tiny hole in my ileum (thelast part of the small intestine) was patched up and an extra layer of MONOCRYL suture sealed the operation successfully.

A Monocryl sutures is a monofilament synthetic absorbable surgical suture. The tiny hole caused peritonitis which is a fatal condition, if not treated. This time a temporary stoma / small opening in the intestines was created to divert the flow of faeces and to let the rest of the intestines to heal. Although I was not fond of the stoma, it was a life saver at that time! I had never seen a stoma nor been in this situation before, so I was pretty annoyed that particular time. That was the first time I was really frustrated and said to The Head of the Department with a very weak voice, since I felt really beaten and weak: "There has been a mistake and I want compensation!"

He commented firmly: "You are not professionals and you should not interfere in these matters. You will not get any penny from this, I can guarantee that! On the contrary, I will see you back in surgery in the next 2–3 years!"

Firstly it was a depressing thought, but it also has had a significant effect on me for life. It was a damn nasty way to say "I am sorry things did not go like they were supposed to!" How do people handle these things when they are alone in a hospital? I don´t know. Luckily, I had my Heli there to fight for my rights, but not everyone has that special someone standing up for them.

If there was one particular time, when I felt both sad and angry, this was it! But the good thing was that I somehow managed to turn that around. It made me so goal-oriented that I decided that I would not return to the hospital if it was up to me! The doctor who operated on me the first time, admitted to me personally, that there was an operational failure and I should have had the compensation, but unfortunately this was the system and there was nothing he could do. I understood him (I had to); he was in a difficult position, but still it was not right.

To be honest, my best compensation has been the strength I got from those Head Surgeon´s words, so I have to say thanks to him. It made me take charge of my life.

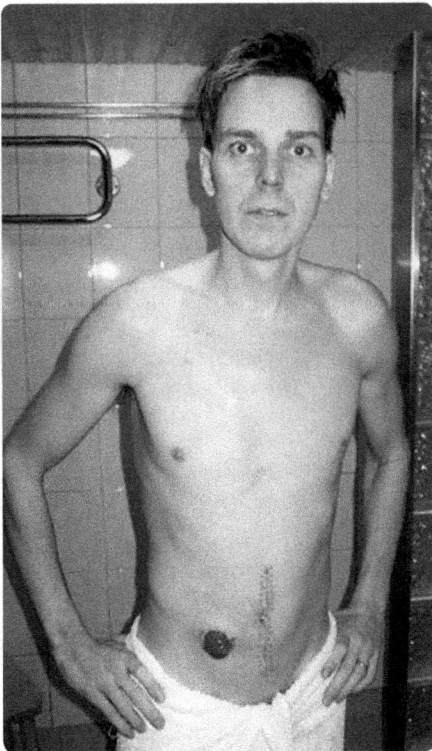

Sometimes when we see a negative thing it can cause positive results! Also, I know there is no doctor who actually wants to fail on purpose and get it on their conscience and onto a failure list. How should the system work so that it can protect both the doctors and patients too?

At that time in February 2004 my weight had dropped to an alarming figure, from around 72 kg / 158 pounds down to 45 kg / 100 pounds, most likely even less than that because I was too weak to stand on some scales. I felt like a skinny Pinocchio with strings – only this time someone else was pulling the strings.

When I returned from the hospital in 2004, my wife had gotten us a dog. Heli said the dog will be my furry therapist and indeed he was! A labrador called Hese. He was quite funny and he was named after a fast-food chain "Hesburger", which is the most successful fastfood chain in Finland. Hese worked in customs as a narcotics dog. He had been in some drug arrests, but he was more famous for getting loose and running off! The day I came home and I went straight to bed, Hese followed and stayed beside me. The bonding started immediately. He had been with us only few weeks and once when we were walking on the beach of a nearby lake, Hese saw a ball on some thin ice and rushed onto the ice. At the same time I knew that very soon he would fall through the weak ice and so I started to walk towards him in the icy water. When I was in the water Hese fell in, but thank God I was there to pick him up from his collar and saved his life. Everything happened very fast, like it was supposed to happen. Sometimes when we act (in the name of love), we do not even know how - it may even be a greater power that is helping us. That was also one of those life-changing moments where you start to see the bigger picture in life!

Hese´s energy was pure light and love which I am and our whole family are forever grateful. RIP Hese. An animal is always a great companion and a healer.

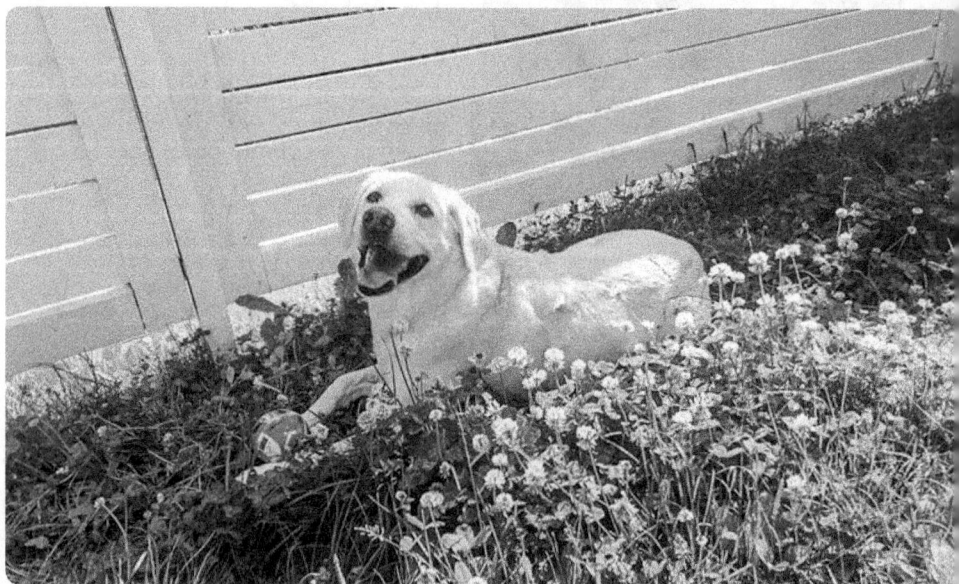

PRECIOUS MOMENTS IN LIFE.
HOWLING TOGETHER WITH OUR
RESCUE-DOG BELLA (2018).

Photo: Marko Airismeri

## MRSA

The Methicillin-Resistant Staphylococcus Aureus (MRSA) infection is caused by a type of staph bacteria that's become resistant to many of the antibiotics used to treat ordinary staph infections. I really hope you can avoid getting an MRSA-infection, because getting rid of it can be a real pain in the belly, which literally happened to me!

After the second operation I was in hospital for weeks, recovering. Something happened that no one could have been prepared for. A fellow patient at the hospital had a seizure and lost his mind. He went crazy one day and decided to rip away all of his cannulas and left his bed shouting, running off and finally falling – landing exactly on my operated stomach.

As you can imagine, it did hurt! I was of course very worried about what may have happened to my stitches and staples. I found out later that he had MRSA and I unluckily got it from him, yikes! Oh my God that was a crazy time! I also had many blockages during the next few months. At that time nothing was moving in my bowel, so it can be quite painful too if the pressure increases. The longest blockage was about 14 days. That time I was just lying on the bed and hoping and waiting for the blockage to release itself again, so that I wouldn't need a third time in surgery. At that time I thought, what the hell will happen next? Will I eventually get out of this hospital alive after all?

In March 2004, an MRSA removal programme was planned for me. That consisted of taking 3 different strong antibiotics at the same time. My intestines had already been bombarded with so many antibiotics before, in between and after the surgery. They were so sore, that I got worried about how much more the intestines could take, and I decided to refuse "any more antibiotics until my intestines were healed again!" I chose an alternative path taking 2–3g of omega-3 daily for several weeks. To my surprise and maybe to the doctors too, I found out that I got rid of MRSA by myself using natural cures such as SCD$^{tm}$-yogurt containing good bacteria, along with honey and omega-3 (1000–2000 mg/day) that may have helped it to go away.

## THE DANGER WITH ANTIBIOTICS

Please do not take antibiotics lightly. Sometimes they can save a life, but in the worst case scenario they can also destroy your life!

The FDA is warning about the use of certain antibiotics (fluoroquinolone) marketed as Cipro, Generic Ciprofloxacin, Levaquin, Avelox, Noroxin and Floxin. It can cause multiple spontaneous tendon and ligament ruptures, spinal degeneration and widespread arthritis etc. I know someone who was perfectly well, but was suffering from a quite normal form of antibiotic-associated diarrhea but it turned into a bacterial infection called Clostridium Difficile. As a result, the person needed constant caretaking. Even single doses of antibiotics for surgical prophylaxis have been associated with an increased risk of C difficile infection. In general, the longer the antibiotic duration and the use of multiple antibiotics (versus a single antibiotic), these are factors that increase the risk of antibiotic-associated C difficile diarrhea.

# CAL-PRO – A TEST TO DETECT INFLAMMATION IN THE INTESTINES

I want to share two good examples regarding Calprotecting levels and how infection levels decreased (from high to moderate level). More about Cal-protecting in IBS-section.

< 50 mg/kg of stool – Negative
50–100 mg/kg of stool – Borderline area. Re-testing needed.
> 100 mg/kg of stool – Positive, may indicate colorectal inflammation

Remember that when giving a sample, it needs to be in refrigerator temperature when stored. It can be stored up to 7 days in refrigerator.

## CAL-PRO 2012

In January 2012 my Cal-pro level was 1700. After an IgG-test I discovered the foods that I am allergic to and I therefore eliminated those foods from my diet for a period of 3–4 months. As a consequence, my Cal-pro numbers went down from 1700 to 400. That was amazing! After a further six months, it went down even more to 130, which was a great number for me. I do not ever remember having such a low figure during my Crohn history and over such a short period.

## CAL-PRO CHARTS 2012

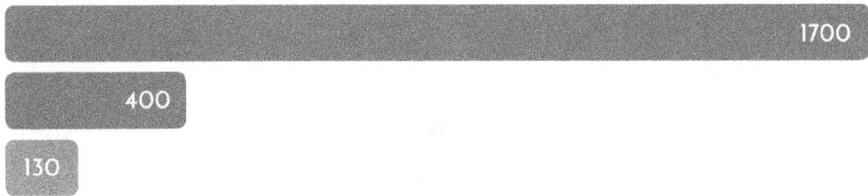

| | |
|---|---|
| | 1700 |
| 400 | |
| 130 | |

## CAL-PRO 2016

In 2016 I drank a smoothie which included carrots. Normally I used just one carrot, but this time I used four and I did not let the juicer do its work properly, which was a mistake. There were still bits of carrots in the drink. The chunks of carrot and the excess fibre created a blockage in my gut, because the next day I suffered from an acute intestinal obstruction(*). I could easily feel the blockage within my large intestine. I massaged it gently with lavender oil every now and then and finally, within about 24 hours the blockage was released. If it had not gone away so quickly, I would have had to go back to the hospital getting fluids. Thankfully, this time I did not need them.

Following that blockage, I had a Cal-pro check within 7 days and it was sky high, 5800! At first it was a huge shock! I had to go back to my healing roots again. I therefore started an acute diet and after two weeks of the first test, the value had dropped back down to 880. It took 11 months finally to get it back down to 200. Patience, a lot of patience is needed with any healing. An elimination diet, olive oil daily (also with enema) and omega-3 supplements all helped me a great deal.

(*) If a blockage takes place; food, fluids, gastric acids and gas build up behind the site of the blockage. If there is enough pressure building up, the intestine can rupture which causes a leak of harmful stomach contents into your abdominal cavity. Early diagnosis and treatment are crucial. Untreated intestinal obstruction can be fatal, so always seek a hospital treatment if you suspect it.

CAL-PRO CHARTS 2016

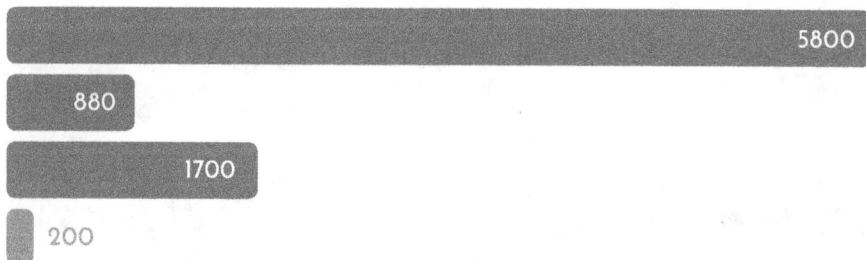

5800

880

1700

200

# COLONOSCOPY

Colonoscopy has been widely used since the 1980's and is the leading diagnostic procedure for colorectal cancer. Colonoscopy is a basic procedure for many patients with intestinal problems. A long, flexible, narrow tube is used with a light and small camera on one end to look inside your rectum and throughout the entire colon. Once the scope has reached the opening to your small intestine, the doctor slowly withdraws it and examines the lining of your large intestine again.

Yet sometimes not going to the hospital for this procedure can be even more of a risk. If symptoms exist, I urge you to go for a check-up.

There is always a risk of a failure. PubMed provided an update on 28 June 2016: "About 2 out of 1000 people who have a colonoscopy have complications that make further treatment necessary. These include severe bleeding, particularly after removal of a polyp, or cardiovascular complications that can be caused by the sedative medications. Intestinal perforations happen in fewer than one out of 1000 examinations. The overall risk of further complications is higher in colonoscopy than in sigmoidoscopy."

You should ask what kind of solution is used to clean the colonoscope; this is a key question that could save your life! Make sure the colonoscope has been sterilized with peracetic acid, to avoid potential transfer of infectious material from previous patients. Widely used glutaraldehyde does not clean the tools as efficiently as peracetic acid. A dirty tool may transfer infections from a previous patient.

## CLEANING THE INTESTINES GENTLY BEFORE COLONOSCOPY

The thing that I do personally is to be a little gentler on my intestines, and so I regularly (few times a year) clean out my own intestines or it can get done by a hydrotherapist, which cleanses it more thoroughly. It is a safe and gentle infusion of water into the colon via the rectum. In addition, no chemicals or drugs are involved and the entire therapy can be both relaxing and effective.

Imagine this: when the intestines are inflamed and so you decide to drink litres / sometimes almost a gallon of the laxative chemical drug that "wipes out and cleanses" the intestines thoroughly before the treatment. What do you think the drug does to your already bruised intestines and its microflora?

Dr. John Bergman talks about colon health in his presentation: "Colonoscopies damage natural intestinal microflora, washing out of the large intestine with large doses of synthetic laxatives, bowel irritation with polyethylene glycol and hypertonic electrolytes. In Crohn's disease the treatment can raise the risk of colon cancer by up to 3200%."

The presentation made me a bit more confident of cleaning naturally.

At least 2–3 days prior to the colonoscopy are the following steps. You can ask for more info from your hydrotherapist.

1. Avoid ALL processed foods
2. Eat probiotic foods like sauerkraut, kefir or goat milk yoghurt
3. Eat apples. Fibre helps with cleansing.
4. Avocado (potassium and magnesium are very important throughout the cleansing process)
5. Sprouted flax seeds (soak and mix well in a blender)
6. Triphala, an Ayurvedic herb
7. Water
8. Probiotics as supplements
9. Peace of mind

Double blind study was done in Northern General Hospital NHS Trust, Sheffield, UK about the effectiveness of topical peppermint oil added to barium sulphate suspension. The addition of peppermint oil to the barium suspension seems to reduce the incidence of colonic spasm during the examination. The technique is simple, safe, cheap and it may lessen the need for intravenous administration of spasmolytic agents. All procedures, especially natural ones that ease the pain for the patient are welcomed.

Dr. Mercola says there are three acceptable screening methods for colon cancer:
1. Fecal occult blood testing (FOBT) done yearly
2. Flexible sigmoidoscopy carried out every five years
3. Colonoscopy every 10 years

# GOODBYE MEDICINE

First of all, let me start by telling you about some good memories that I have about medicine. Sadly, there are not many. Remicade (which is an intravenous-ly-given biological medicine) has helped me few times (especially in 2008), it was actually the first medicine that had really helped me, even though it was just for a short period of time. Sadly, its use had to be stopped after three treatments because of its side effects. It gave me an almost 'immediate' feeling of suffocation and chronic allergic symptoms on my skin, which I'm still recovering from today in 2018. In rare instances, some patients suffered central nervous system disorders, including the confusion of immune system responses that inflamed and decayed blood vessels. In America, Remicade side effects have even resulted in blood disorder lawsuits. Many times taking a drug is like walking on a long tight rope across a steep mountain in foggy weather without knowing what is on the other side.

March 2004 was an important time for me, for it was when I finally decided to open my eyes to the synthetic world of medication. I did not find any good reason to stay on this path any longer. I felt like I had a once in a lifetime chance and almost felt obliged to try something else while the rest of my intestines were recovering, thanks to the stoma.

From that month onwards, I decided that I would try and treat Crohn's disease in the best way that I could. This time I allowed more time for natural healing, still leaving a door open for synthetic medicine should there be a new cure. I started by turning many things upside down. Not taking the medication that was not helping and changing my diet by being very selective with all food. They were huge changes to be made, but this time I was very determined!

First I had to reject hospital food. Easier said than done, but I did it. I ate some of it but very selectively. No more bread (gluten), white sugar or processed meals. That was the first step. I was really struggling of course with the phenomenal transformation. At the same time I was lucky to have had so much help with the diet my wife and I found, the Specific Carbohydrate Diet ™. SCD™-food was a big help in the beginning. My wife helped me to live SCD™-lifestyle. Especially useful was the home-made 24H-probiotic yogurt, which I ate for two years between 2004 and 2006. My wife Heli, my mother, grandmother and my aunt all made and helped to prepare and store the yogurt. I am therefore so very grateful to all the women in our family who helped me return to good health from my sickbed!

When you sell something, isn't it normal that you should truly believe in and even be prepared to use the product yourself before you can sell it to customers?

Doctors have a huge burden on their shoulders when they are dealing with toxic treatments. A study was done that involved 1081 doctors at Stanford Hospital which asked what doctors would do if they had to choose an aggressive treatment to use on themselves. Is it a surprise that most doctors (88%) would turn down the option of aggressive and toxic treatment such as chemotherapy if they were terminally ill, yet still they are recommending it to their patients?

Dr. VJ Periyakoil, who is a Clinical Associate Professor of Medicine at Stanford University School of Medicine, believes the problem is that the medical system rewards doctors for prescribing medicine and taking action, not for talking with their patients to find out their real issues. Modern cancer centers are now integrating palliative care and delivering it at the very same time as cancer treatment.

# AND THE HEALING STARTED
# – RECOVERY TOOK 2 LONG YEARS

I have never been skinnier than I was in 2004, I have never been overweight, but when my weight went under 100 pounds / 45 kg it really hit me! My life was a total disaster at that moment and it was hard to find the way out. I often thought about giving up. I was not living the life I had dreamed of. It felt like someone else had taken charge. Everything was off course in my life at that time. Later on I learned to accept it and I realized that it all had great significance in my life – ever greater than I could ever have expected.

I was practically a skeleton and I had no idea about my future. My family and friends were supporting me in every way possible for which I will always be very thankful. I remember when my friends Jari, Japi and Harri brought a light sword to the hospital for me. We were joking "Luke, be aware, I will rise again." Thank you guys! Humor and staying positive helped me enormously.

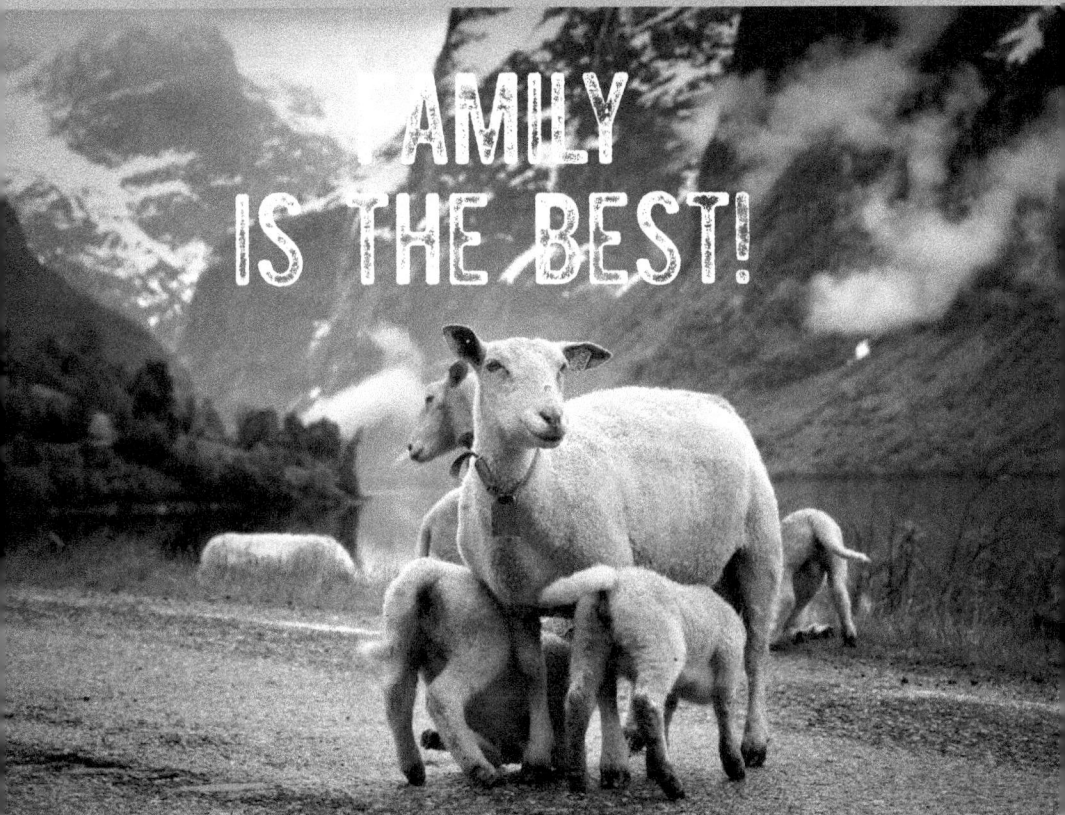
FAMILY
IS THE BEST!

The most important and positive person in my life is my beloved Heli. She always kept me on a positive track and literally helped me to cope and survive. I am forever grateful for her love and for keeping my head up and for guiding me through the process. I do not know what would have happened to me without her love ♡. But indeed my mother and my stepdad Martin were a huge help too! I really felt loved! It is amazing how it helps to talk to people. I did not belong to any support groups, but I felt how the burden became easier whenever I met and talked to different people. One day in 2004 Jehovah Witnesses visited me and talked with me. Although I have a different vision about spiritual beliefs, talking with them helped me a great deal back then. I thank them too. What I mean is that the help can come from different people, from people who you would not expect it to come across. Talking with someone you do not know can be very therapeutic. The worst thing is to stay indoors and see no one and wait for the depression to hit like a tsunami. I had to fight against it, because it was not easy but very doable anyway!

I had one thing very clear in my mind, I had decided to do everything that I could on my part to be healthy again. If I had to get rid of unhealthy food choices, I would do so. However this is always easier said than done. How can you say "no" to chocolate bars when your mind craves for it? When I gave up my chocolate temptations for a month and then I took two bites of chocolate, you know what happened? The same day, my intestines started bleeding. It was that serious for me! If I wanted to stay healthy, I had no other choice than to change, big time! (to quit chocolate, sugary sweets, burgers, bread etc. for a certain period of time at least). That restrictive period lasted for two years. Today now that I am in much better health, my intestines can take a small amount of sweet foods. But my habits have changed also into much healthier choices.

To be honest, I totally brainwashed myself when it came to sugar consumption. I no longer have huge sugar cravings. Heli has made homemade fudge and I make homemade raw chocolate sometimes. But I have quit white sugar completely and I use alternative sweeteners like honey and organic raw cane sugar, BUT in moderate amounts. The great thing when eating raw and natural sweeteners or sweet food is that the amounts are way smaller compared to factory made chocolates. Because I already know the consequences, my guilt kicks in early telling me when to stop. It is a great thing too that organic snacks are getting much more popular in stores today, so some bars are OK to eat.

# DIET HAS A ROLE IN MY RECOVERY

To know what is best to eat with this condition can be the easiest or the trickiest part. If you are a city person, it might be tricky because today our food is so overly-processed and full of chemicals. Living in a countryside can give you more options to organic food choices.

A very important thing is to learn that you are the key in finding the right things for your own wellbeing. I am sure you will need to let go some of the old habits that are not good for you. When changing something, the first thing you need to do is to step out from your (old) comfort zone and leave behind the habits that are not good for you, gradually, step-by-step. Don't expect that everything will happen overnight. Give yourself time and especially, be gentle on yourself.

I was literally out on the cliff-edge when I made those changes, so I had to jump out of my comfort zone practically in one day. I am sure my athlete background helped me hugely in making that decision! This time I was not going to track and field competitions, but for something more permanent. The goal was much higher than breaking one record.

When I started my soft training and healing journey back in 2004 it was 100% SCD™, especially 24h-yoghurt (half of the yoghurt was cream in order to get some fat around my bones) which was boosted with extra probiotics, honey and some ripe bananas and blueberries. For lunch, I had a gentle carrot soup, oh my God – my food was so simple back then (and boring), but it was well worth it and so important for healing!

After a period of 3 months I started using other fermented products too. There are many to choose from ie. kefir and sauerkraut. There are also plenty of fermented juices to choose from for example Kombucha (fermented tea), mead (fermented honey), water kefir and dairy kefir from coconut milk for starters. The best thing is that you can make these at home or buy them from the health stores. Thank God for health stores and for the kind and warm-hearted people working there! The best stores are those with bio organic fruits/vegetables and even nuts that are fermented. You can also try sour pickles or kimchi (Korean spicy pickled cabbage).

TODAY: Today my diet consists of a combination of different diets like the SCD<sup>tm</sup>-diet/ Paleo/vegetarian/mediterranean (red meat in my diet is almost non-existent), plant-based diet and lots of different smoothies with healthy oils. My diet now contains many more options than the strict SCD<sup>tm</sup>-diet I had started with, but I am so thankful that the diet existed. No more white food (sugar, flour, salt, processed and refined food).

You will find more detailed information in "Tools for healing-section".

## TOMMI´S KEY POINTS

- Decision to heal myself
- New diet
- Anti-inflammatory smoothie with healthy oils daily is my nutritional lifeline!
- Restoring beneficial bacteria
- Diagnosing food allergies (igG)
- Using as little chemicals as possible, favoring organic in everything. Especially in food and personal hygiene products (using natural mineral stone, organic toothpaste, organic cosmetic, lotions etc.).
- Loving myself
- Loving family
- Spending time in nature
- Hobbies, travelling, friends
- Rest and sleep
- Love conquers all

# I WANT TO THRIVE, NOT ONLY TO SURVIVE!

# MONEY AND SOCIAL SECURITY

What if I say that I have saved hundreds of thousands of dollars by making better choices and being healthier, would you listen more carefully? If you are an IBD patient, you'll know that fifteen years without having any medical aid, surgeries, medicines etc. you'll be saving a fortune. That is what has happened to me.

Let´s face the facts. We need money on a daily basis and money runs society. We have built our society so that success and sickness seldom go hand-in-hand.

Money takes up a huge part of our daily lives. Yet, money should be the last thing we should worry about, especially when we are sick, but unfortunately it seems to be the opposite. We value too many things in life that are based simply on making money and on profits – that is one of the reasons why our society is so greedy and lost today.

In Finland we have a good social security system that could be a model to many nations. Finland enjoys one of the world's most advanced and comprehensive welfare systems, that's designed to guarantee dignity and decent living conditions for all of its citizens.

It pays most of our medical expenses, but we also pay high taxes here to make such a great system possible.

We used to say that it is like winning the lottery to live in Finland. With today's rising expenses it feels like you need to win the lottery to be able to live well in today's society!

The Finnish social system is challenged every year and it is not the same as it used to be, but it is still pretty good. I wonder how long we can keep the system going, especially now when we are facing so many different crises around the world. Having to experience the Greek financial crisis and the ever-growing refugee crisis within Europe at the same time? They are a common burden to all EU countries.

We also really need to take a closer look at rising medical expenses. These crisis moments have good sides to them too because people learn to depend on each other again and are more willing to help others.

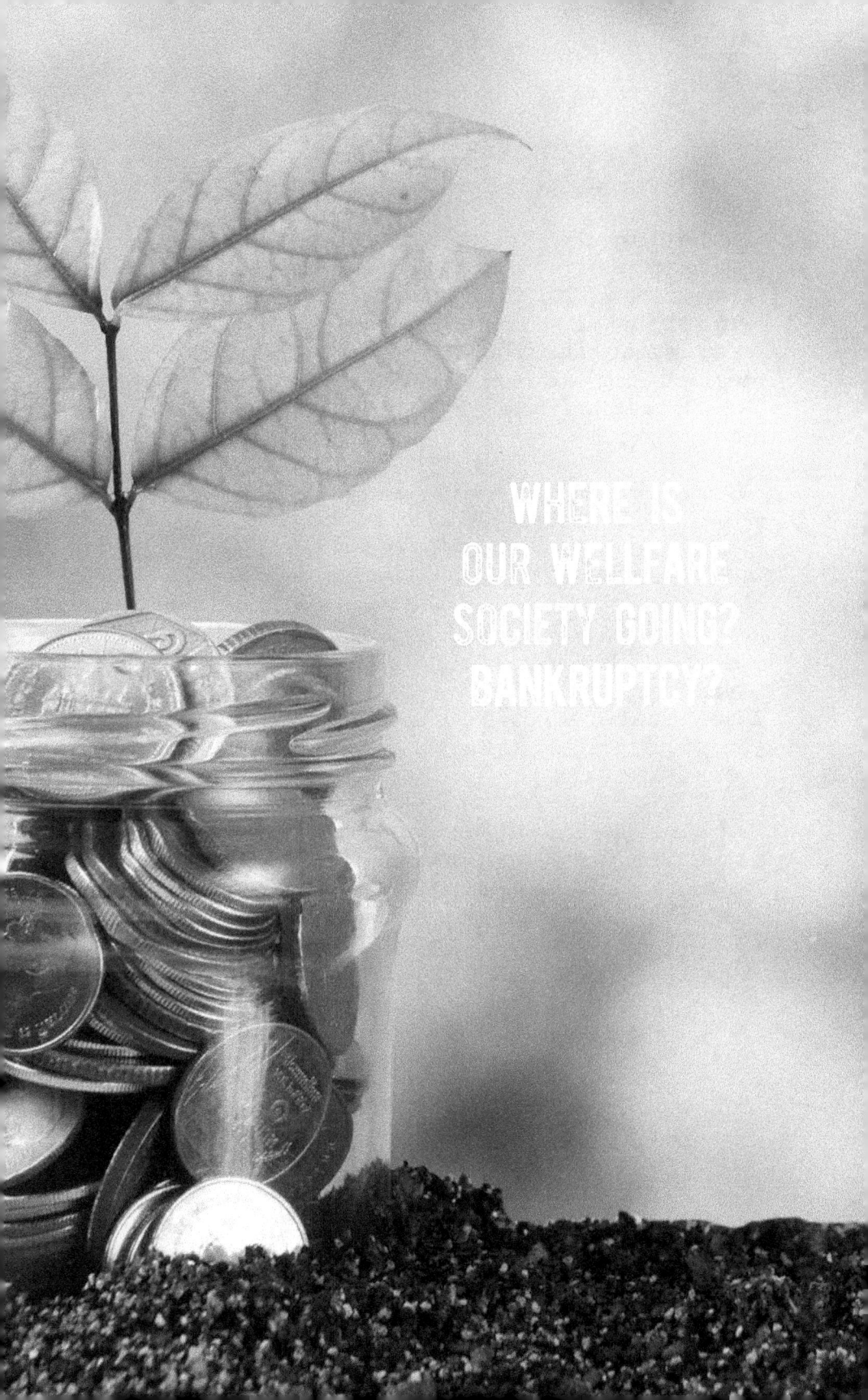

WHERE IS
OUR WELLFARE
SOCIETY GOING?
BANKRUPTCY?

# BEING HEALTHY SAVES YOU A FORTUNE!

I calculated roughly how much money is required to treat my IBD. By not using medicine and being in a good shape for close to fifteen years now, I have saved our society well over 200,000 Euros for not being sick. See "Medicine prices in Finland 2015" (p. 128). Although this is an estimation and it depends on how you calculate it, the main thing is that I feel so much better today! It is amazing how huge the difference is between being healthy and sick. A huge improvement in my medical expenses has also been that there have been NO surgeries or operations since 2004.

I was offered many different expensive medicines for treating my Crohn's, for instance:
• Humira injection pen (8 ml), 1200 € (two shots every month)
• Remicade, 2500–3000 €/dose. Given every other month.

Here are two other examples of typical medicine treatment costs (USA):
1. Statins, a simple cholesterol medicine in America is priced at $14,600 USD a year.
2. One single pill for hepatitis C virus costs $1,000 USD. A 12-week course of Sovaldi costs $84,000. Even with Medicaid coverage, patients are set back about $600 USD a pill.

The fact is that it is extremely expensive to be sick. It is such a profitable business too for the Pharmaceutical Industry because through constant 'conditioning' by our doctors and the media, we are blind to believe in one solution only – and that single solution is synthetic medicine.

> I HAVE SAVED OVER 200.000 € BY BEING HEALTHY.
> IT IS THE BEST DEAL OF MY LIFE!

# THE WAY WE LIVE TODAY

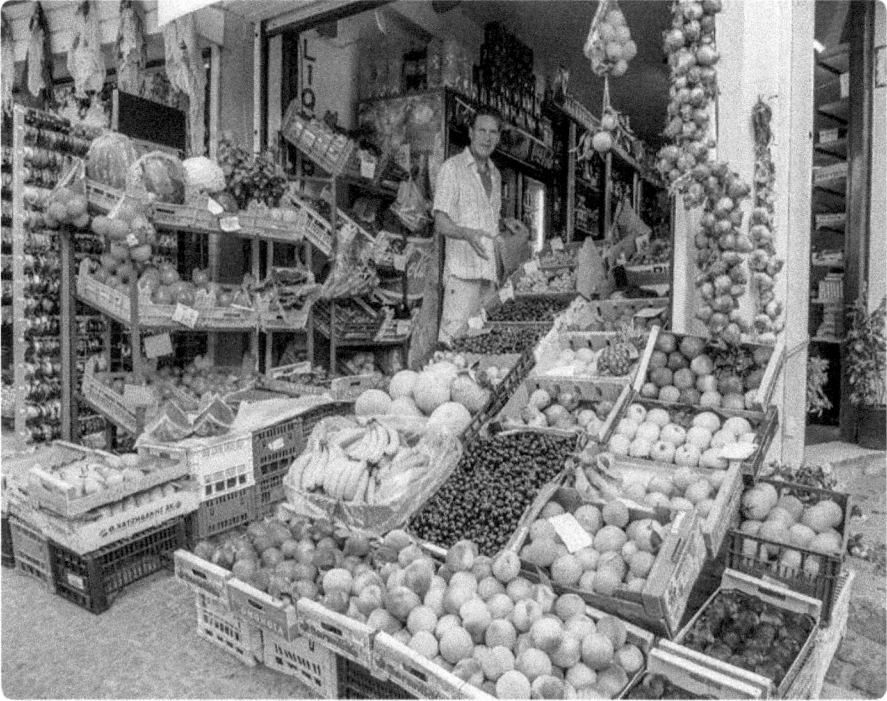

*Once upon a time all food was organic.*

If we think about the food we eat today, to simplify, it can either harm or heal us, depending on the choices we make. I strongly recommend that you treat your gut well, with love and pay attention to your symptoms. Your body will tell you if something is wrong, so all symptoms are important to take note of.
The most natural choice is to eat organic food to prevent gut diseases, but of course it's not as simple as that. So what does 'eating healthy' mean? That is a little more complicated in today's world because we have so many choices to choose from.

Gluten for instance can hide in your body showing quite visible symptoms like: gas, abdominal pain or cramping, bloating, diarrhea or constipation and Keratosis Pilaris otherwise known as chicken skin, is a skin condition that appears as elevated, hard bumps on the skin. They look like red goosebumps, but they stay on your skin. This skin condition along with dermatitis herpetiformis, a similar skin condition, has been linked to gluten intolerance. It can also appear as a mental illness, mood swings, chronic fatigue or even infertility. Try to live gluten-free life for 3 months and see if you feel any difference.

> WHEN BLAMING GLUTEN, REMEMBER THAT GASTROINTESTINAL SYMPTOMS OF DIFFERENT DISORDERS MIMIC ONE ANOTHER. THE GUILTY ONE CAN BE SOMETHING ELSE THAN GLUTEN. WHAT YOU FEEL INSIDE MAY BE THE TIP OF THE ICEBERG.

Do tests as Blood-, endoscopic-, stool-, breathtests etc. and they may tell you the real reason. Also check your medication for side effects.

Is diet a significant source of pesticide exposure in young children? Recent organic diet intervention studies suggest that it is. These studies have focused on children living in suburban communities. An organic diet is knowingly associated with reduced urinary concentrations of non-specific dimethyl OP insecticide metabolites and the herbicide containing 2,4-D in children.

Although the test was pretty short, they got amazing results with reductions of 49% in pesticide exposure when the children ate organic food. They collected urine samples over 16 consecutive days from children who consumed 'conventionally-grown' food for 4 days, organic food for 7 days, and then conventionally-grown food for a further 5 days.

The easy conclusion to make is that we should go back to the old times when pesticides were not used. Yet we have a growing population needing more and more food. What also can be seen is the shift towards vegetarian choices because factory meat production is a huge burden on our planet.

# 3 GOOD REASONS TO WAKE UP

## POOR DIET KILLS MORE THAN SMOKING

A poor diet contributes to 1 in 5 deaths globally. Unhealthy eating kills more people than smoking. Obesity was revealed to be the fastest growing cause of death in the world. A study by the Global Burden of Diseases (GBD), published in The Lancet.

## SMOKING ADDICTS AND KILLS

"Smoking kills an average 1,200 Americans daily. Secondhand smoke kills over 38,000 Americans each year. Children exposed to secondhand smoke are at an increased risk for sudden infant death syndrome, severe asthma, and reduced lung function. Nicotine `changes the brain,´ which makes it hard to quit smoking. More people die every year from smoking than from murder, AIDS, suicide, drugs, car crashes, and alcohol combined."

## MORE OBESE CHILDREN THAN EVER

World will have more obese children and adolescents than underweight by 2022, if current trends in food marketing, policies and pricing continue as they are today. We need stronger laws to protect children from unhealthy foods. A study by Imperial College London and WHO.

*Photo: Sanna Kostamo*

# FOR THE LOVE OF SPORTS

This story is also about not giving up and above all else – having a love for sport! The ability to move and do exercises has constantly kept me motivated to be as healthy as possible and do the things I like most.

I have always been keen on sports and it has given me a lot. It has been my way of emptying my head from stressful situations and I am forever thankful for every moment it has given me and also kept my body in good shape. When I was a teenager, I had a great chance of doing track and field sports in Kaarina, Finland. It provided me with great friends, a good physical condition. but also coordination that allowed me to learn other sports.

It is good to try and do many different sports when you are young. Team sports are great and very popular, but if you want to surprise your (hockey/football) team mates with explosive body weight movements and an athletic ability, martial arts are the perfect addition. It also gives you different kind of discipline which can help you throughout life. Gymnastics is also excellent if you want to be a versatile athlete. Although I am already an 'old fart', I still enjoy many different sports like ice-hockey, badminton, gym, floorball, free diving, rowing etc.

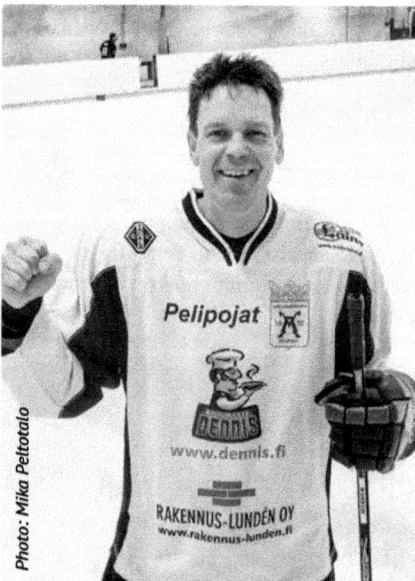

Photo: Mika Peltotalo

for

Although I love doing sports I also love helping others. I have been privileged to be the sports manager the ultra-sportsman Markku Saarinen. Our greatest event so far has been the world record (unofficial) for indoor cycling in Lahti, Finland in 2013. Markku cycled amazing 2798 miles / 4503 km in 7 days with only 2–3 hours' sleep at night. The distance equalled the trip from Finland through Europe and all the way to Casablanca, Morocco.

I have had great moments in my sports career, but when you can help someone else, it is even greater.

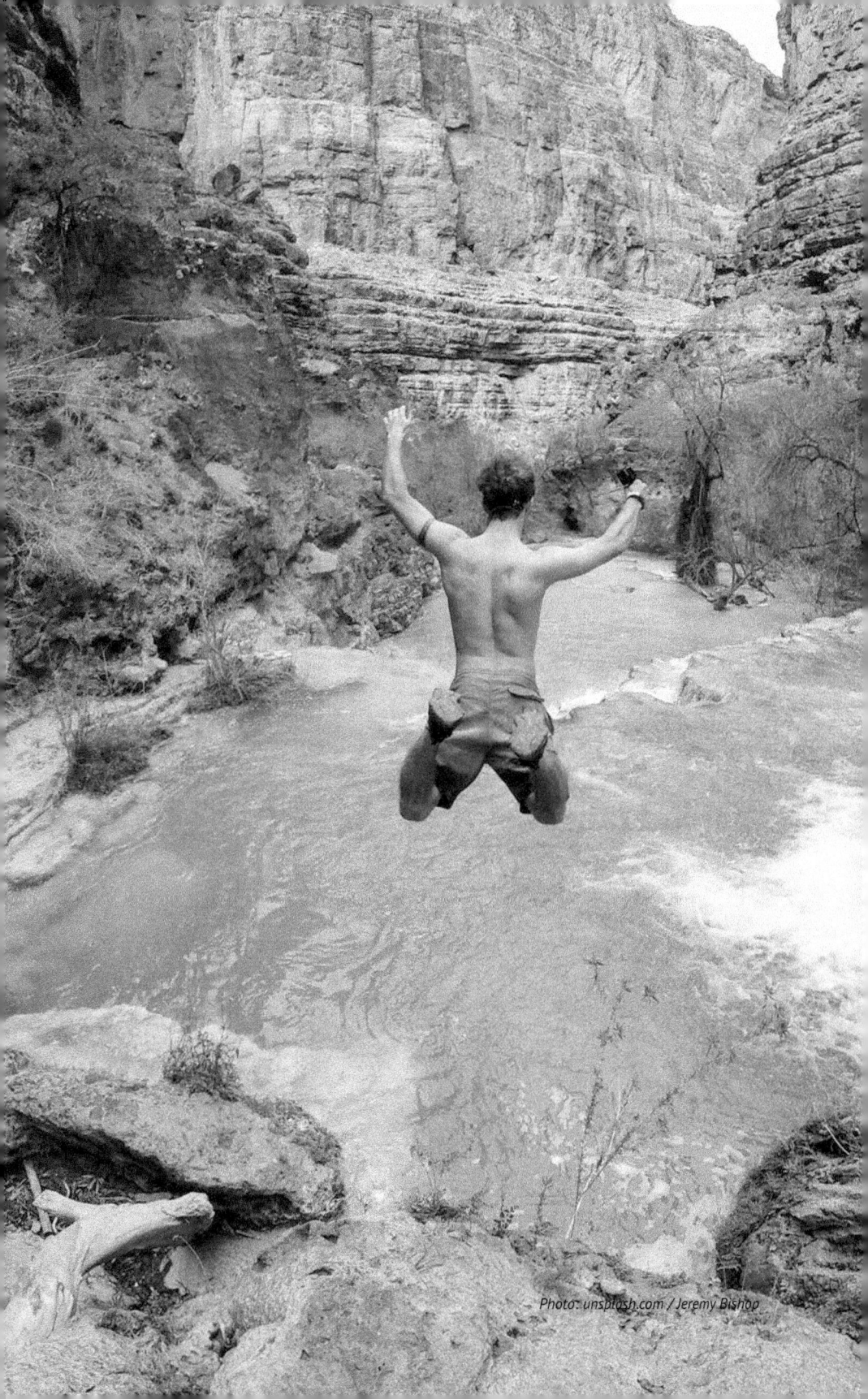

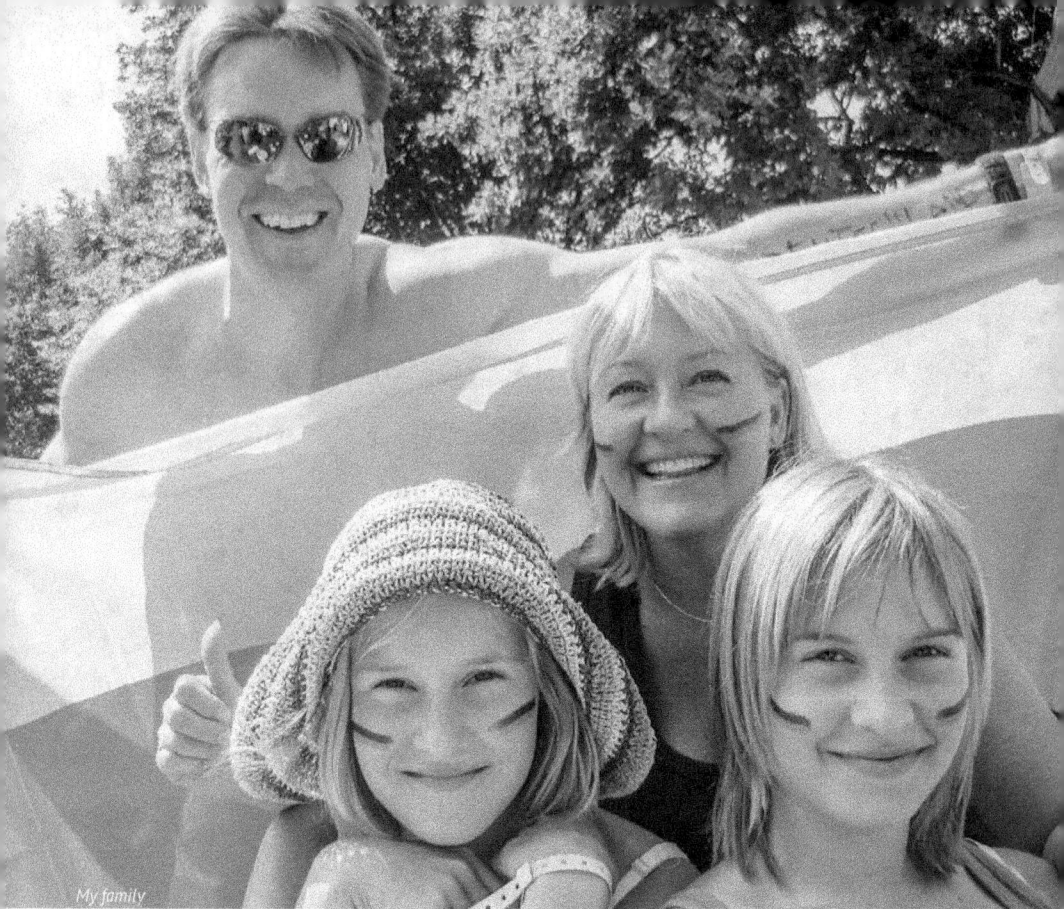
My family

## TRAVELLING WITH IBD

Leaving home with someone who has to deal with gastrointestinal problems or having uncontrollable diarrhea, is not easy, and so going on an airplane can be an extreme act. Travelling has been a huge concern to me because it has always been important for me to see the world. My situation was so bad in the year of 2000, that my doctor did not suggest any trips abroad. I started to think about what to do, fear the worst or just go for it. I decided to GO FOR IT! And I have to admit that I was totally crazy (about travelling)!

> MAY YOUR CHOICES REFLECT YOUR HOPES.
> NOT YOUR FEARS.
> NELSON MANDELA

For me, travelling has been yet another inspiration and motivation to be healthy again. It opens up new perspectives and helps to understand and deal with different situations in our daily lives. In addition to seeing new places, it creates friendships that last a lifetime. I simply love travelling! Travelling is often done with someone very special and I have to say that I would not have been travelling so much if it was not for my beloved wife Heli. We have visited more than 30 countries so far.

Despite the disease, I have managed to travel to many places so here are some tips that I have found that are useful, and also some extra information about different locations.

# FLORIDA – THE SUNSHINE STATE

## SUNBURN

The USA has left its huge mark on me, I love the country and its people. Every time I go back, it feels like I'm going home.

Oh, how I adore Florida and the warmth! Especially because we live in such a cold climate in Finland, so we really appreciate the warm weather. At least for vacations. The humidity is very high and of course that has its own challenges. Here is a great natural healing tip that we discovered in Florida, while canoeing in the Manatee River and getting sunburned (despite the commercial sun lotion we used): we bought an Aloe Vera plant, sliced its leaf and applied its translucent gel - the liquid natural gel the plant produces, generously to all over our sunburned area. The next morning the pain was all gone and our sunburn had been healed! Miraculous stuff indeed!

Tip: Mineral sunscreens are safer than chemical sunscreens. Mineral sunscreens are also more effective the moment they are applied, unlike chemical sunscreens which require approximately 30 minutes to become effective after application.

How do you avoid (seeing and visiting) fastfood chains in the USA? Mission impossible. Almost on every corner there is a deli, pizza place or some kind of a chain restaurant. During our visit, we were mainly eating healthy homemade food cooked by our friends, so thankfully I knew most of the time what I was eating. Occasionally during the daytime we stopped at fast-food restaurants when the children were hungry. Oh boy was that a mistake… Well, for me it was! It may sound weird, but I was fascinated back then about seeing how well my intestines could tolerate fast food again. I tried it once at each of the traditional chains like McDonald's (Big Mac), Burger King (Double Whopper), Taco Bell (Burritos) and a donut by Dunkin Donuts. The scent of a fresh donut is amazing, I must admit, but the donut itself is so very treacherous for my intestines.

After one week I started getting symptoms like itching etc. After two weeks my intestines started to bleed. Back in Finland four weeks later, I was forced to go to the hospital because the bleeding did not stop. My intestine was examined, and it was found to be in a very bad shape and thoroughly infected and ulcerated. I had to undergo Remicade treatment, a biological and very expensive drug. It helped me at the time, the bleeding stopped, however using the Remicade had to be stopped after few times because of the strong side-effects of taking the drug (skin disorders and choking feeling).

I learned on that trip that some of the additives used in foods can cause big problems to sensitive stomachs like mine. Emulsifiers like "Polysorbate 80 and carboxymethylcellulose" for instance need to be avoided at all costs.

I was back on the natural path again, searching for alternative solutions. I instinctively knew I had no choice but to try my best to prevent the sickness in the first place. The healthy road continued with even more motivation after this trip.

GREAT IN FLORIDA: Nature, animals, people, sunshine, fruit, organic food stores

BE AWARE: Fast and processed foods

# EGYPT – LAND OF PHARAOH´S
# AND THEIR REVENGE :)

If you ever get the chance, please go and see the Pyramids. They should be visited at least once in a lifetime. Every time I see them I wonder how those stones had been moved to their locations? It is easier to believe that a higher intelligence presence was involved there, how else would it have been possible to move them?

For me, Egypt has been a mystery in many ways, but also with regards to my gut health. In the River Nile, in the area around Cairo, the chronic disease Bilharzia is commonly found which is caused by the water being infected with blood flukes or parasitic worms that live in fresh water in subtropical and tropical regions. If you get this infection, you may need to take Praziquantel, a prescription medication, for up to 6–8 weeks after the trip.

We absolutely love snorkelling and free-diving and so far the best place for us has been the Red Sea, especially the town of Sharm El Sheikh. Our dream is to go to Marsa Alam, much further in the south and close to the Sudan border, which is considered to be an almost pristine place for diving and snorkelling.

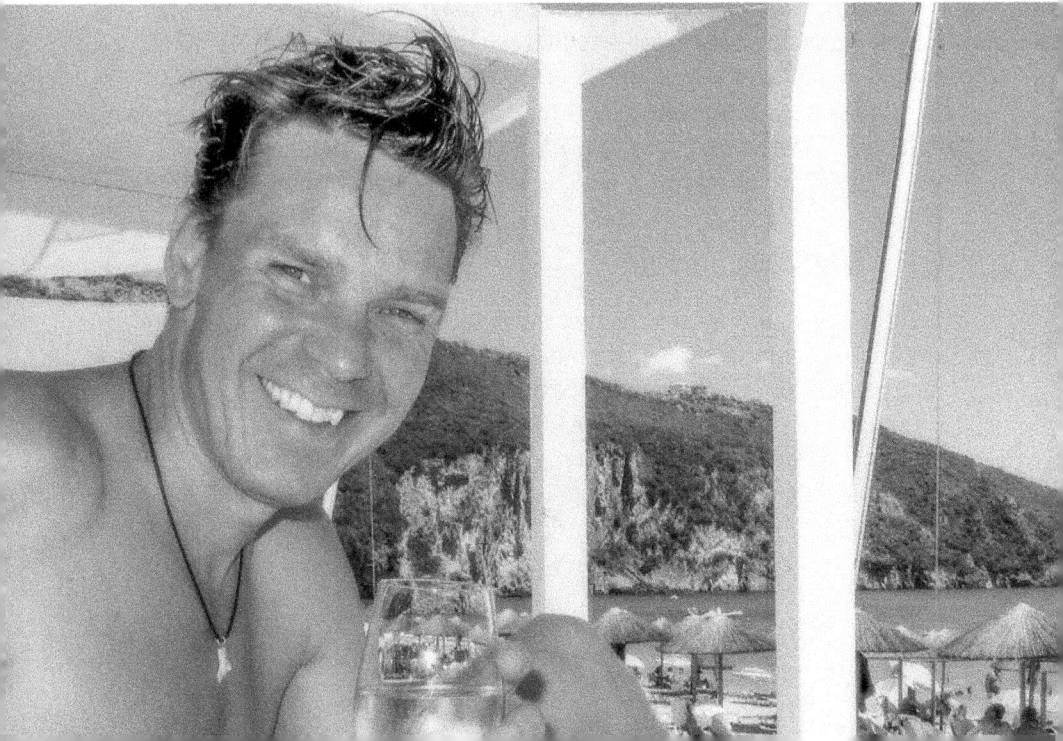

We have visited Egypt 8 times, staying at many 3-star to 5-star hotels. Guess how many times I have had diarrhea? Answer: 8 times. The reason can be in restaurant hygiene, that gives food and drinking water the problematic bacteria.

I have been searching for ways of how to clean drinking water. I found out that E. coli bacteria can easily be killed by some herbs and spices, so it solves one small part of the problem.

Good herbs and spices to use are: garlic, clove, cinnamon, oregano or sage. I sometimes even add a hint of baking soda or pure sodium bicarbonate (½ teaspoon) to 1 liter of water to make the Ph-level a little higher, making it a body cleanser. When going on a vacation, your own stress mechanism in the body may allow stress-related flu or cold to develop. Baking soda is capable of fighting cold and flu symptoms in your body.

Two scientists from the National Environment Engineering Research Institute (NEERI), in Nagpur India have proved that clove oil has a strong antibacterial agent that can transform unclean, foul smelling and alkaline well water into clean and sweet water with "favourable mineral qualities."

Twice I have been hospitalized in Egypt, getting fluids for rehydration in Sharm El Sheikh. I am sure you are wondering why on earth I keep on going back to Egypt? The simple answer is that we have not found a better place for freediving and snorkelling within a reasonable flight time (5 hrs) from Helsinki. I am actually amazed at the fact that coral reefs in the Red Sea even beat "the paradise on earth", the fabulous Similan Islands in Thailand, which are considered to be one of the best diving sites in the world. Gosh, when you look below the sea, sadly you will realize how fast our nature is being destroyed, also in Egypt.

## DIARRHEA WHILE TRAVELLING

Diarrhea can happen to anyone and thankfully it can disappear in a day or so with proper attention. My situation has always been a little bit trickier because of IBD. It does not take long for your body to lose fluids and electrolytes. I have been in a situation where there was no doctor available and so I needed additional fluids. I was drinking as much fluid as I could, which was simply not enough. So I had to figure out what else I could do to get hydrated.
The solution? I had a warm bath for about an hour and I added some sea salt and about 200 grams of organic, vitamin-rich raw cane sugar to the water. It was the

exact same drink that I had been drinking to get hydrated, but this time I let it absorb through my skin. Thus I was treating my dehydration both internally and externally, and it solved the problem!

GREAT IN EGYPT: History, architecture, ocean life, the local people.

BE AWARE: Different strains of bacteria and the local water, eating fish especially from the Nile may contain bilharzia, so anything that you eat, even cooked food or food washed in fresh water might upset your stomach. Tap water in general contains very different bacteria levels than we are used to. Do not brush your teeth with tap water either. Clean all water with clove or other herbs and spices.

FOOD: Eat only cooked food to minimize any contamination from bacteria. Salads, ice-cream, egg and milk products get contaminated easily in the heat.

HYGIENE: This varies greatly from our point of view, so keep some hand sanitizer with you at all times.

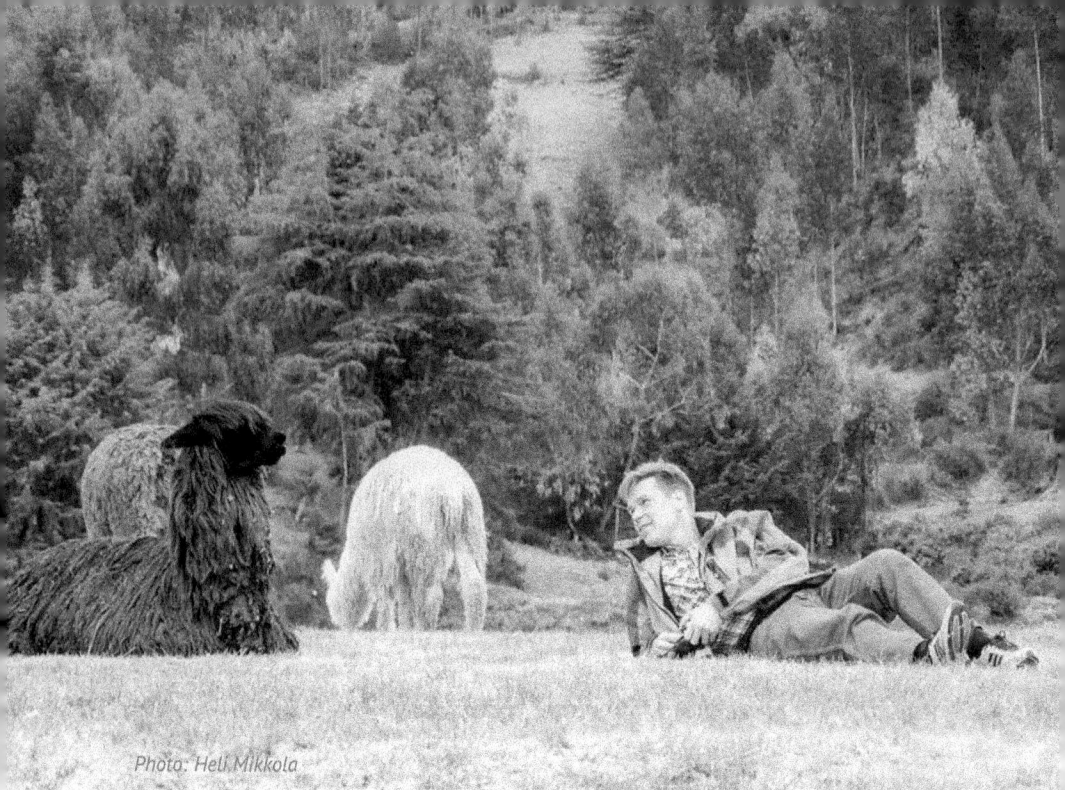
Photo: Heli Mikkola

# PERU – THE MOST MAGICAL PLACE IN SOUTH AMERICA

Every place is unique, but Peru is something purely magical, with its ancient history and architecture dating back to the ancient Incas and even pre-Incas as well, it's truly an astonishing culture. I recommend Peru with all of my heart. Please bear in mind that the high altitude may give you difficulties, so allow yourself at least 3-4 days to get used to the different altitude, drink lots of water and avoid any alcohol or tobacco products. Coca plant leafs are used widely and legally for mountain sickness. I also learned that cannabis is a wonder plant for many illnesses. Lawmakers in Peru have voted in favour of a bill to legalize medical marijuana, allowing cannabis oil to be locally produced, imported and sold. It is now the sixth country in Latin America to legalize the use of cannabis in some form.

Cusco, the old capital of the Incas, is located at 11.500 feet (3.500 m) above sea level. Cusco is the gateway to the sacred valley of the Incas, into the amazing Machu Picchu, ancient city of the Inca royalty, miraculously built on top of the mountain.

THE NAKED GUT

## THE BEST BREAKFAST

Close to our accommodation was a tiny restaurant that was so easy to fall in love with. My favorite breakfast was a simple smoothie containing:
- real mango
- plenty of lucuma powder
- water

The drink offers vitamins, protein and antioxidants that protect the body against colon, breast and prostate cancers. While it does contain the mellow sweetness of lucuma, it's low on the glycemic scale and typically suitable for diabetics.

## DURING FLIGHT - EXERCISE AND DRINK WATER – NO MORE FOOT SWELLING

The flight to Lima from Helsinki is something that needs real planning. It took over 30 hours including stopovers (Helsinki-Stockholm, Sweden-Frankfurt, Germany-New York, USA-Texas, USA-Lima, Peru). On the way over to New York I drank about 500 ml of water every hour and no alcohol, naturally. I chose vegetarian meals for easier digestion. I managed to do about 1000 squats (seriously!) in the airplane, in front of the water machine, and it worked like magic! I had no problems whatsoever with my stomach, swollen ankles or headache - symptoms I normally would have had with long flights. This is a simple yet highly effective recommendation!

When I had the chance to decide how to travel from Lima to Cuzco, (Cuzco is a convenient place to go to in order to see Machu Picchu) either by bus or by airplane, that was an easy choice. 21 hours versus 1,5 hours. The bus takes you through the Andes mountains, which would offer you stunning scenery during the day time, but sitting and sleeping in the bus for 21 hours was not an option for me. It was not at all tempting, especially after the long flight hours to get to Peru.

In Peru it was great to see that people still use quinoa rather than grain flour to bake. Gluten-free quinoa is used in many places, especially in Cusco. Quinoa is used daily in foods and desserts.

Chocolate Chip Cookies are baked with a mixture of quinoa flour and brown rice flour. They are sweetened with coconut sugar and an extra bonus is that they use coconut oil too. They don't use any eggs, just so you know that you can bake delicious cookies without using eggs. What a better way to eat sweet food than this? So, no worries even if you can no longer eat grain flour or refined sugar. There are so many other great alternatives too, totally nutritious and healthy, simple recipes which are actually easier to make!

## CHICKEN AND ANTIBIOTICS

One particular warning that many locals, including tourist guides in Lima kept telling us was "Do not eat Peruvian chicken. They are fed lots of antibiotics and fattened up in just a few weeks for the restaurants".

Later on I found this old and dusty article: "Ministerial Resolution prohibiting the importation and sale of hormones for fattening poultry. - 13.IX.1960 - El Peruano, No. 5822, 16.IX.1960, p.1: Prohibits the importation and the sale in Peru, of oestrogenic hormones for this purpose." So, at least the problem has been noted. Whether it is valid and is being controlled or not is another story.

## A FOOD CHAIN IS GOING ANTIBIOTIC-FREE

In 2016, the big Fast-Food Chain 'Subway' went Antibiotic-Free - and not just for chicken.

When you are travelling in rainforest areas like the Amazon, be aware that there are many small animals that can make your trip a real adventure. My wife went to see the shore of the River Urubamba in the village of Aquas Calientes, close to Machu Picchu. She sat on the rocks just for few minutes and got bitten 200 times by mosquitoes! They got infected and caused her feet to swell severely. Thankfully, antibiotics and mountain salt baths worked that time. It's good to remember to protect and cover yourself while in the jungle area!

What also upsets your stomach is getting robbed. If it is only material things you lose they can always be replaced, but health is another matter. However, having your things stolen is upsetting. In Peru many people warned us about pickpocketing. It is amazing how easily it can happen. One of the group members, let me call her Rita, was having breakfast in a nice hotel, in downtown Lima, in an area that is said to be the best and safest there is. Rita was sitting in the chair and waiting for the others and put her bag on the floor next to her seat. Next thing we heard was that her bag had been stolen in front of her eyes. We saw from the surveillance camera that a stranger from outside came into the hotel with a huge backpack. He just walked by the reception, and headed straight down the stairs to the breakfast room. It looked as if he was nervous, looking for a table, he walked through the room and saw the bag on the floor. He kicked the bag up off the floor and into the air for few feet and then grabbed it from there, and while walking back up the stairs he put it in his backpack. The whole episode took about 40 seconds. Boom! That happened even faster than getting sick from bad food. Rita lost her valuables, some of her clothes, camera and all of her money which ruined her day both mentally and physically. Luckily she was travelling with a group of generous people, so they collected enough money for her to continue the journey.

## CLIMBING AND HEALTHY EATING GO HAND-IN-HAND

What I saw in Peru when combining hiking and eating healthy food was a real eye opener. When you hike, you should only use the natural, healthy ingredients that your digestion system can easily absorb and handle. That way our digestion does not have to do all the extra hard work that it has to do with processed foods. Especially when you're hiking - avoid all processed food and alcohol. Drink clean water. Hiking itself is hard enough for your body at those heights, so do not make it any harder by fueling yourself with harmful food or liquid.

So why not do this every day – hiking or not!

> In general; do not eat empty calories like white bread, fast foods, artificially sweetened sodas, energy drinks, sugary candies and other processed foods. For a snack, choose wholesome ingredients that you already know by their names, like honey, sesame seeds, cashews, almonds, avocados, apples etc. This way your body does not have to do extra work to transform the food you eat into a nutrient-rich fuel for your precious cells. You will gain extra advantage and benefits by eating healthy and organic food too.

GREAT IN PERU: History, people, ancient knowledge, landscape, delicious and healthy food. Peru has great varieties of organic cacao, Creole is one of the most famous one. Peruvian raw chocolate is super-healthy and delicious.

BE AWARE IN PERU: Altitude sickness and pickpocketing.

WATER: Drink bottled water only and make sure the cap and seal are still on when you buy it.

FOOD: Go for local food. Watch out for chicken, it is raised using hormones and antibiotics. Eat cooked food to minimize any bacterial infection. Salads, ice cream and milk products get contaminated easily, so watch out for those.

HYGIENE: Use hand sanitizers, especially after handling money. Use soap and water too.

CLOTHES: Cover yourself with protective clothes to avoid mosquito bites etc.

PICKPOCKETING: Keep your valuables in a safe place and do not carry all your money in one place.

ALTITUDE: Prepare yourself by drinking a lot of pure water, chew coca leaves that are present everywhere in Peru. If you want an extra tip – improve your VO2 max levels – this is the maximum volume of oxygen that a body can use – which will allow you to absorb even more oxygen. Using an elevation training mask before the trip can be extremely useful too. Any time you climb above 8000 feet/ 2400 m, you run the risk of suffering from altitude sickness. While the ultimate goal is to keep this illness away entirely, it's good to know the signs in advance. The most common symptoms include headache, nausea, fatigue, dizziness and sleep problems. More serious effects include fever, dry cough, brain swelling, and other complications.

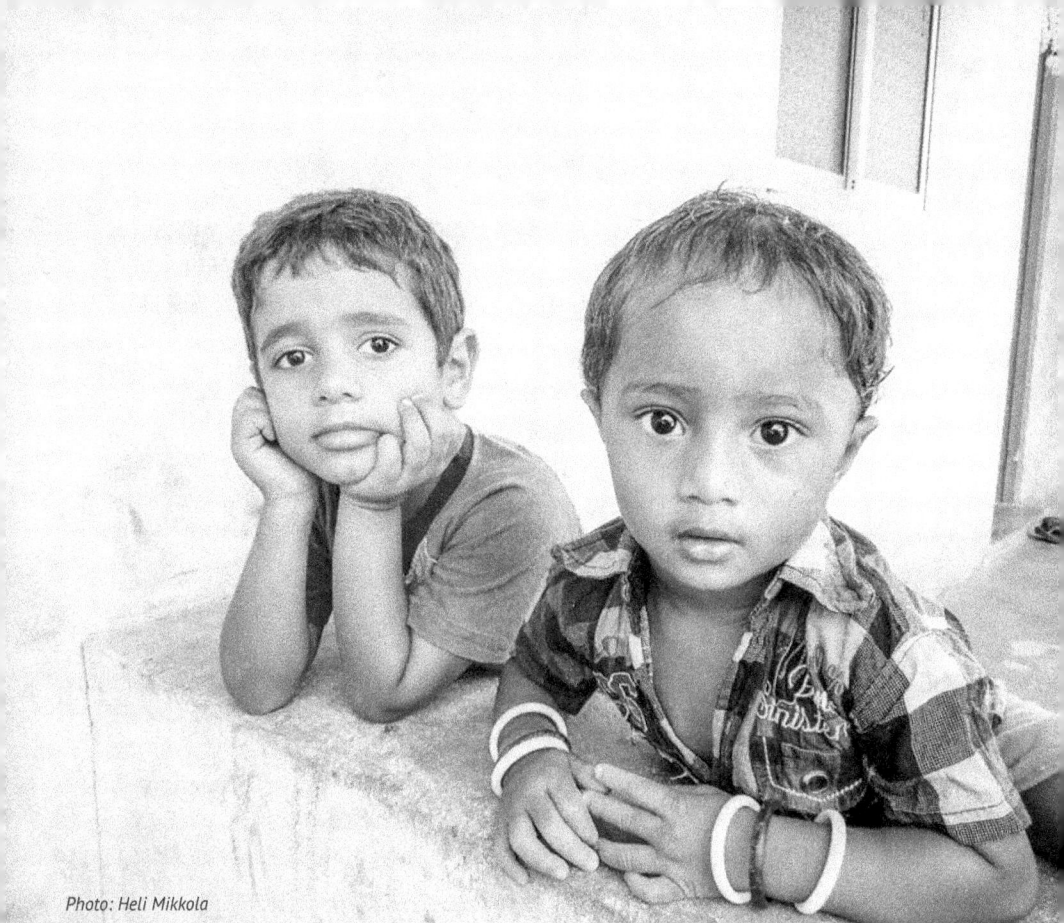
Photo: Heli Mikkola

## ADVENTURE IN INDIA

Exotic India, there is something enchanting and mesmerizing about this beautiful country that attracts people from all over the world. Amazingly lush countryside, a fabulous animal kingdom, friendly people and such delicious food, to name but a few. India is also a country full of contradictions and with over a billion residents, India has the highest number of people living below the poverty line, which leads to much lower hygiene standards than we are used to. Be aware that India has many local bacteria and viruses that your immune system would never have encountered before. Food in India is amazingly cheap according to our standards, so avoid buying foods from really cheap restaurants & food stalls on the streets. These vendors often have very little understanding about hygiene and cannot afford to throw away food unless it is really rotten and they often have no access to safe water. So, just go to the more expensive restaurants where the dinner will still cost only about US $2.00 – 4.00 / €3.00 Euros.

Rice, fruits, coconut and cooked vegetables, and fresh fish from the local fisherman have so far been our safest choices. Do not eat raw vegetables, because they might be washed in water that is not safe enough. If you get them served to you in restaurants as a side dish, just leave them on your plate. If you like to eat fresh vegetables, buy them yourself, rinse them with mineral water and preferably buy those that you can peel before eating, it's the same thing with fruits. Buy fruits that can be peeled, like lichees, bananas, mangoes, apples, oranges etc. Avoid drinking fresh juices pressed on the street like sugar cane juices. We have seen the fresh juice stations using water from a drain by the roadside to clean their machines, enough said? :)

If you can get over these obstacles, India has many of the nicest people in the world. Their hospitality, such as that at Albert's in Morjim in Goa, takes us back again and again. The humble Nepalese people have also won our hearts; Jimmy, Pawan, Tapan, Madhav etc. have all left their marks in our hearts.

So far, I have not been sick in India from food ever, but I have managed to get self-inflicted diarrhea there. What I did was something unthinkable. I had a massage at the beach in Goa. A perfect way to relax under the shade, listening to the waves, half asleep...

After the treatment I was thirsty, and grabbed the first water bottle I saw, taking a sip out of it. The masseuse yelled "NO, DO NOT DRINK IT! It's tap water, which I used to flush your feet!"

I spat it out of my mouth, it was there for few seconds only. I even put hand sanitizer in my mouth and gargled with it, to minimize the damage. Thank God I did not swallow it. Had I done so, I probably would not be writing this book now. The mouth is a very sensitive, fast absorbing area, and I literally have proof of it. Within a few hours, my stomach got really sick, with immense pain, and I not only got diarrhea but I vomited fiercely. It took a few hours to cleanse my gut thoroughly! It was all over after one day, so I was very lucky that time.

We have been so blessed in our travels so many times. We have visited national parks, fed wild monkeys with bananas, taken care of stray dogs and even elephants within sanctuary areas, and of course we used a lot of hand sanitizer. It is a huge blessing to be able to do those things without getting sick. We look forward to the next adventure and so we still want to be on the safe side when it comes to hygiene.

I normally rent a scooter on our holidays to get around more easily. With a scooter, you can feel the air and see more than you would do just by walking. Tapan, one of our hotel staff members in Goa in India asked me to give him a ride to a shop nearby to buy some shampoo. "Of course, let´s go", I said. That moment something changed inside of me. Heli and I both took 400 ml (13,5 OZ) bottles of shampoo with us for our 2 week holiday. I must admit, I could use much less.

After we rode to the kiosk and Tapan bought his shampoo, when he explained how he uses it, it really opened my heart and soul... Tapan bought one single sachet, containing 2 ml (0,06 OZ) and said "That will last me 1-2 weeks and I will wash myself and my clothes together the same time." Very convenient!

Sachets generate huge amounts of sales in India. Most of the shampoo sales are through single use sachets. What this means is that it is much easier to sell 50 sachets than 1 bottle. Quick turnover means lower costs. Sachets are primarily sold through smaller retailers who again run with lower margins and overheads. Bottles are often sold through supermarkets with higher overheads.

This occasion made me question the way we live our lives by over-consuming the planet's resources. Our worlds may be different concerning the way we live, but we still share the same passion, love and joy for life. I eternally thank you Tapan for opening my eyes. I love and respect you very much!

GREAT IN INDIA: Delicious, healthy vegetarian diet, sun-ripened fruits, sunsets, friendly people, beautiful scenery, warm ocean water, sunshine, animals, plant kingdom

BE AWARE: Strong sun rays, hygiene, take extra caution with fresh water. Always drink bottled water (cap sealed). Keep hand sanitizer handy at all times!

# GREECE – THE LAND OF GODS AND GODDESSES

Greece is most definitely one of our favorite places despite the financial crisis and migration problem they presently have. Beautiful scenery, food and culture bring us back again and again to this mighty country. It's a country where you can live on mainly olive oil, tomato, cucumber, onion and feta cheese. No wonder Mediterranean cuisine has been chosen to be one of the healthiest in the world. The traditional Mediterranean diet has shown it may reduce our risk in developing conditions like type 2 diabetes, high blood pressure and raised cholesterol, which are all risk factors for heart disease. Researchers have also found that people who closely follow a Mediterranean diet may live a longer life and be less likely to put on weight.

## WHAT MAKES GREEK FOOD SO HEALTHY?

A typical Greek diet includes lots of vegetables, fruit, fish, beef and lamb (moussaka, stifado). A good thing that you do not find in the Greek diet is processed foods. I would like to point out at least two favorite Greek foods that are consumed in large amounts.

**1. Feta cheese** (sheep's milk or a mixture 30% of goat's and 70% sheep's milk) which makes it a good choice if you have problems digesting bovine dairy products. Over 12 kg per person of feta is consumed yearly in Greece. Feta cheese is lower in fat and calories than many other types of cheese. A one-ounce (28g) serving has 4 grams of protein and only 74 calories. Strong flavor means you can get away with using less cheese without feeling cheated. Processed foods on the contrary often have sugar and additives that change the taste and make you eat more. It has been said that feta has even cancer-protective effects. Calcium is an important mineral for the prevention of osteoporosis, colon cancer, and the regulation of blood pressure. Phosphorus and Vitamin A are essential nutrients that can help protect and even enhance your vision.

## 2. Olive oil – the healing oil

- Rich in antioxidants (vitamin E, vitamin K)
- Reduces bad cholesterol (LDL)
- Raises good cholesterol (HDL)
- Lowers blood pressure
- Contains chemicals that help prevent cancer and ageing
- Thins the blood
- Guards against diabetes. An olive oil rich diet is not only a good alternative in the treatment of diabetes; it may also help to prevent or delay the onset of the disease.
- Helps the digestive system
- Dark chocolate with Extra Virgin Olive Oil improves cardiovascular risk profile (University of Pisa)

A greek friend to our parents, Georgios said already in 1970´s "Eat olive oil, it will keep you healthy".

**Annual consumption of olive oil in Greece: 17,9 litres. North America and Northern Europe consumption is rated around 0.7 liters a year.**

As knowledge increases about the health benefits of olive oil, the use of this amazing oil has been rising rapidly in all countries around the world. Especially in Asia where until now people did not know about the beneficial health properties of olive oil as a food, as they have considered it to be more of a pharmaceutical and cosmetic product. Olive oil is the only vegetable oil that can be consumed as it is –freshly pressed from the fruit.

TIP! DEHYDRATION AND HEAT STROKE

One day when we were in Greece, our daughter was playing at the beach, in direct sunlight, forgetting to drink enough water and to cover her head. She got sick and started to vomit as a result of dehydration and heat stroke. A doctor holidaying next to us rushed up to help: he grabbed ice from the nearby tavern, placed it within a towel, and pushed it gently onto our daughter's neck. He said it will quickly lower the body temperature and restore her strength. He also brought us a large glass of mineral water, stating she needs more minerals in her body after vomiting. Plain water will not replenish important minerals when you are exposed to such hot temperatures. This is good to keep in mind when vacationing in hot countries.

# HANDY ALL-AROUND TRAVEL TIPS

1. DURING THE FLIGHT: Keep moving and drink lots of water. Avoid alcohol, it dehydrates your body.

2. EAT COOKED FOOD: When possible have your meals cooked to avoid harmful bacteria. Avoid fast food and additives by reading the labels on your food purchases, and also by being extra careful when eating out in a restaurant.

3. SAFE SNACKS: Make your own or buy natural food snacks (nuts etc.)

4. WATER: Drink plenty and purify your water (clove etc.) The quality of water served on an aircraft may not always be the best, so it may be better to buy your water in bottles in the duty free and take it on board with you. Make your own beverages instead of buying sugary sodas.

5. HYGIENE: Take good care of hand hygiene. When going to the bathroom start by washing your hands FIRST with soap. You need to clean your hands every time you handle money. Keep hand sanitizer available at all times.

6. SUNBURN: Coconut oil is good and natural but the protection won't last long. Avoid sunburn also by wearing clothes and staying in the shade rather than putting chemicals (sunscreen) onto your skin. According to the Environmental Working Group (EWG) approximately 75% of commercial sunscreens contain toxic chemicals that are linked to cancer and also disrupt hormones. There are sunshine tablets (astaxanthin etc.) for preparing your skin and preventing sunburn. If you get sunburned, use Aloe Vera.

7. DAY RHYTHM: Try to keep the body's rhythm as normal as possible. Take naps and use melatonin to help you alleviate jet lag. Melatonin has strong antioxidant effects. Preliminary evidence suggests that it may help strengthen the immune system. The strongest desire for sleep or sleep drive (internal circadian biological clock) of adults generally occurs between 2.00 AM – 4.00 AM and in the afternoon between 1.00 PM – 3.00 PM, depending on whether you are a "morning person" or an "evening person."

8. USE PROBIOTICS: These are your gut-vitamins. If you're going to be traveling, take Saccharomyces boulardii (yeast probiotic) a few weeks before your trip. It may help prevent traveler's diarrhea which usually comes from ingesting food or water that's been contaminated with bacteria.

9. FIBER: Dietary fiber, found mainly in fruits, vegetables, whole grains and legumes, is probably best known for its ability to prevent or relieve constipation or diarrhea.

10. BE AWARE OF THE LOCATION OF THE CLOSEST TOILET: For knowing that gives you piece of mind. Keep extra toilet paper in your bag, always.

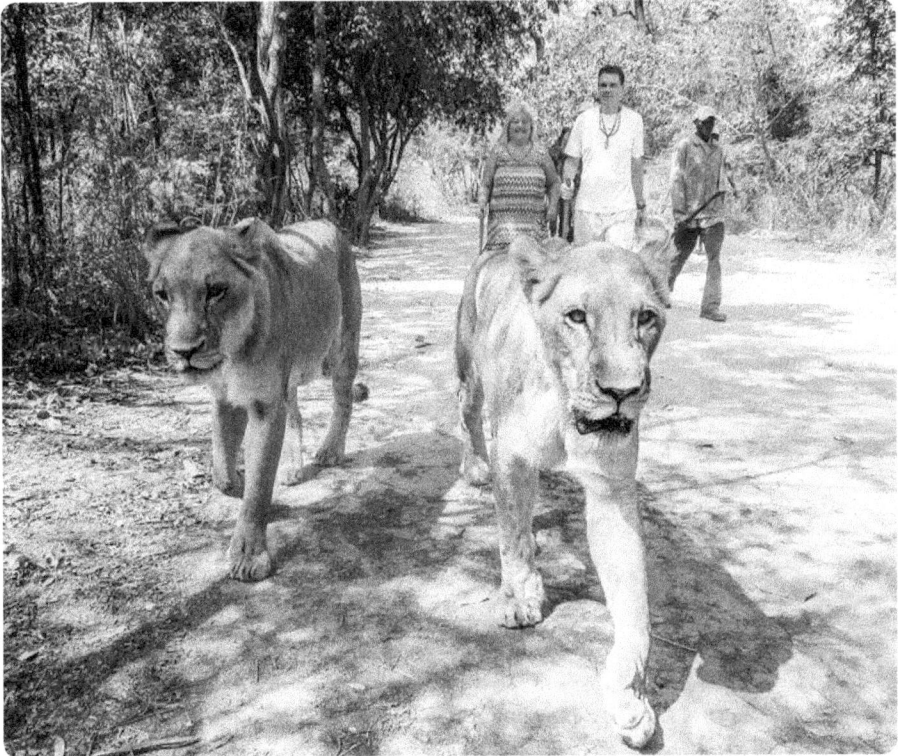

# EASY TRAVEL FOOD

Gluten free tortilla
by Vani Hari, Foodbabe.com

Add safe toppings that you can handle.
Mustard (choose sugar free), avocado, lettuce,
red pepper, pickles, carrot (shredded).

Cover the tortilla in greaseproof paper
and put it in a sandwich bag.

How convenient!

# EASY TRAVEL DRINK

33 / 1 L oz of Water
Pinch of quality salt
1-2 teaspoon
of raw cane sugar
1 teaspoon of
organic apple cider vinegar

While flying, you can take the ingredients with you in a shaker and
then mix them with a bottle of water which you'll need to buy in
the airplane. Rehydration is the key in preventing many (digestive)
problems. And by the way, alcohol is not a rehydration drink :)

# EASY IMMUNE BOOSTING FOODS

Want to boost your immunity while travelling?
You can find these foods almost everywhere:

### 1. GARLIC
Fights against: Viruses and influenza

### 2. HONEY
Organic and locally-grown
Fights against: Bacterial infections, candida infection.
It also coats the linings of the stomach.

### 3. APPLE
Organic
Great for: diarrhea, insulin resistance,
allergies, Staphylococcal infection

### 4. TURMERIC
Spice it up with black pepper to boost the effect
Treats: oxidative stress, inflammation

### 5. SALT
Himalayan or unrefined sea salt
Great for: Maintaining fluid balance, preventing dehydration,
relaxing muscles and treating low blood pressure. Reduces the risk
of infection and kills harmful bacteria.

Staying hydrated is one of the easiest, simplest ways to stay
regular when on the road or in the air. Water, coconut water or
herbal tea are great choices.

# TOOLS FOR HEALING

The idea is to show you some of the
cornerstones in my healing path in the last
15 years and present them to you. Use a
professional guidance, take controlled steps
and get better and long lasting results.

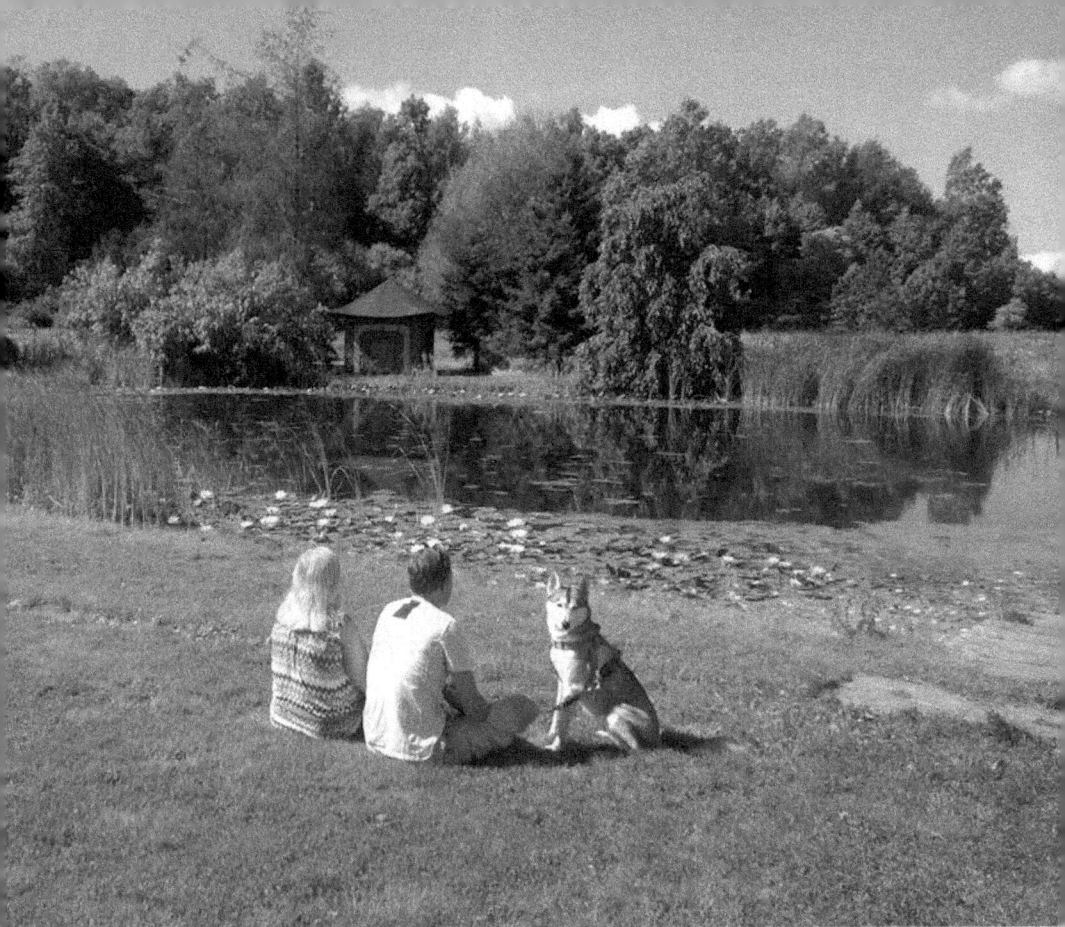

# 1. MIND

JESUS SAID: "BECAUSE YOU HAVE SO LITTLE FAITH.
TRULY I TELL YOU, IF YOU HAVE FAITH AS SMALL AS
A MUSTARD SEED, YOU CAN SAY TO THIS MOUNTAIN,
'MOVE FROM HERE TO THERE,' AND IT WILL MOVE.
NOTHING WILL BE IMPOSSIBLE FOR YOU."

Your body's ability to heal yourself is much stronger than anyone has permitted you to believe.

The mind is a very powerful tool in many ways. It is our most valuable asset. When you believe in yourself, your mind will give you powers that can move mountains. I warmly suggest that you put effort to work on your mind and let it be your healer. I have witnessed the mind being ones best friend, but also ones worst nightmare too many times.

When I decided in my mind that I would heal myself, that was the first step towards a much more positive and richer life. That path and learning, is of course an on-going and a lifelong endeavor. The more you learn to love and appreciate your body, the more your body loves you back.

Between 2003–2004, when I was not able to do any exercise for over one year, I had already started doing imagery training from my hospital bed. This mental rehearsal made me visualize myself as a healthy patient doing all kind of sports, especially track and field which I used to do it when I was competing in my 20's, so it was easy to start doing it again. I was able to visualize, feel, and sometimes even smell the grass from the track. It felt just like I had never stopped doing it. Anyway, those simple practises done on a daily basis helped me to stay motivated and to greatly improve my wellbeing along the way. I felt that the visualization had helped the healing process move along more quickly than just lying in bed waiting for the miracle to happen. I practiced this every day to take my mind away from the sickness.

It is so important to take care of your physical body, but if your only goal is to look good from the outside using the phrase to appear as "hard as a rock", your body will wake you up sooner rather than later.

The real strength comes from the inside. When both physical and mental aspects are in balance, that is when you truly rock!

The older and smarter you get, the faster you will notice the importance of our mental capacity. Start your day with a smile and see "the sunshine", every day. Seek a positive companion where ever you are. Positive people give you energy instead of stealing it.

Easy exercises that educate your mind are like silk on your body. Yoga, meditation and Tai Chi are great examples. Also, as we all know it very well, being in nature is super-healing.

An animal can be a great companion and a healer too. Studies have shown that when owners interact with their dogs, the human and the dog appear to release oxytocin ("gratification hormone"). It is the hormone your brain releases when we love and care about someone. It's a funny thing, but it has also been shown that dogs' oxytocin levels get 5x higher than cats. Still, lots of people have long believed in the healing power of cats. Either way, they are great companions! (a study conducted for the BBC TV show "Dogs Vs Cats").

## 2. DETOX

Getting your body clean and healthy can result in a wide range of positive effects. **Number 1 reason is to remove toxins from the body.** Long-term exposure to toxins (environmental pollutants, chemicals, preservatives, pesticides, heavy metals, and industrial waste for starters) affects our metabolism, behavior, immune system, and eventually they all lead to disease. They are stored in tissues and cells throughout the body, not only in the colon. Detoxing helps our systems function properly again.

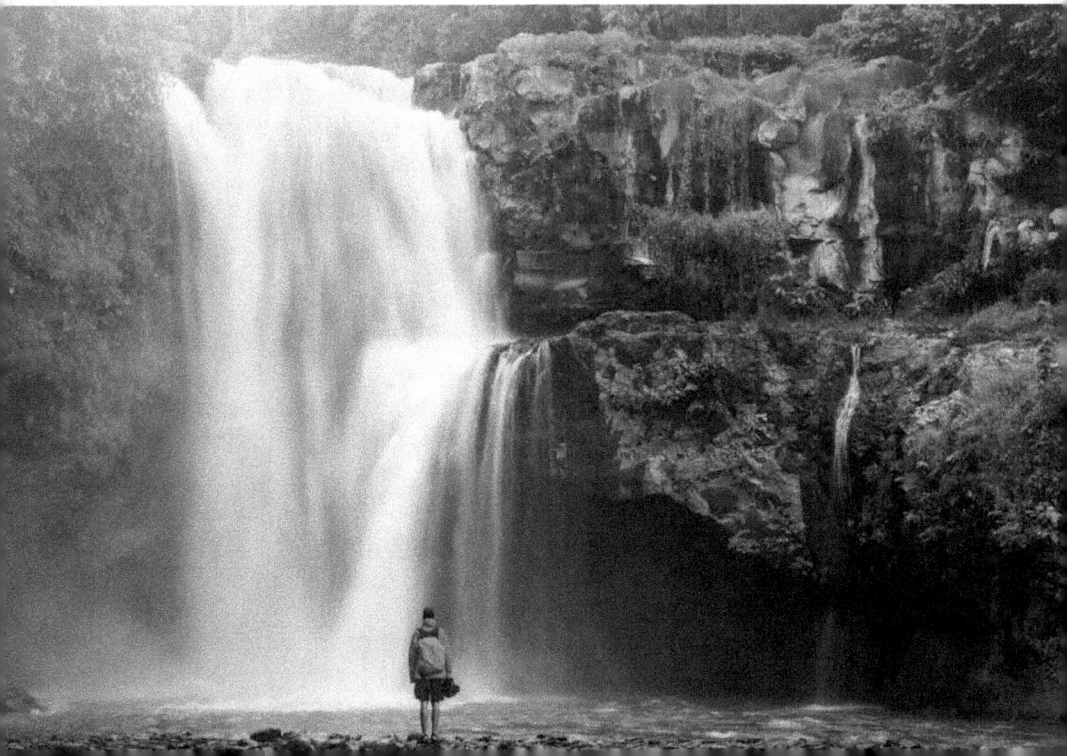

# 10 DAY FASTING

## IN THE MORNING

A. Start your day with a 17 oz / 0,5 L of water with one squeezed lemon.
   Add 1 spoonful of extra virgin olive oil.
B. 15 – 30 minutes later have a smoothie

**Ingredients:**
1       cucumber (or watermelon)
4       celery stalks
2       apples
6 – 8   leaves kale (Tuscan cabbage) or spinach, red chard, parsley etc.
        (the darker the leaf, the healthier they are)
1/2     lemon
1 inch/ piece of fresh ginger (easy way to peel ginger is to use spoon as a 2.5cm
"knife", that way you do not waste too much of this golden treasure)
        You can alter the recipe and add greens like Chlorella or Spirulina

## LUNCH

C. Steamed vegetables and brown, organic rice. For dessert some berries.
D. In the afternoon, enjoy tomato-, beetroot- or carrotjuices or something
   similar with berries. If you feel cold, drink herbal teas.

## DINNER

E. Enough smoothie to keep you going.

After the ´detoxing´ period (5 – 7 days) you can add some texture by adding
banana, avocado, mango, pineapple and some honey. Just make sure you are not
allergic to any of these. After 10 days finish the detox and feel vibrant! :)

Avoid sugar, artificial sweeteners, coffee, dairy products, red meat, alcohol,
processed foods, oils like vegetable oil, canola oil, soybean oil, and of course
anything hydrogenated or partially hydrogenated. Wheat, gluten and white rice.

There might be decades of built-up toxins, especially if you have never done it before. An enema or a professionally done colon cleansing can have a significance effect on your health. After all, the colon is where approximately 90% of the digestion and absorption of food occurs, so in order to keep it in good condition you need to clean it regularly.

Please note: When the colon is inflamed, be cautious, even with water. So that it does not further inflame the colon.

All you need for an enema or a colonic irrigation is:
• An enema bag with a plastic tip (from pharmacy)
• 2–4 L / a gallon of lukewarm, clean water. Buy a water filter that removes impurities by minimizing the contamination of water using a fine physical barrier! Don't use tap water!
• (for example, chlorine kills good bacteria). Use spring, filtered or still mineral water (not carbonated). Do not use distilled water in order to avoid electrolyte imbalance. You may add 1 to 4 tablespoons of organic apple cider vinegar into the enema bag. It has vitamins and probiotics that are good for you!
• 30–60 minutes in the toilet
• The colonic cleanse must be done step-by-step, and very slowly to avoid damaging the intestinal lining
• Use olive oil to lubricate the tip

**Using essential oils in gut health – Consult with a professional aromatherapist to avoid any misuse. Use only 100% pure, organic essential oils**

## CUMIN EXTRACT FOR IMPROVING IBS SYMPTOMS

Symptom Control in Patients with Irritable Bowel Syndrome is a study by Tehran University of Medical Sciences. Cumin was taken 20 drops a day orally. It was shown that cumin extract can be effective in improving all IBS symptoms. Abdominal pain, bloating, incomplete defecation, fecal urgency and presence of mucus discharge in stool were statistically significantly decreased during and after treatment with Cumin extract.

## SITTING IN THE RIGHT POSITION IN TOILET

Make things easier in the toilet: The Asian 'squat' is better, it relaxes and straightens the rectum, while our "westernized" version of going to toilet and sitting makes our rectum more tense. The least you can do is buy a product like squatty potty or make your own version of it. The Asian squat will make your elimination faster, easier and more complete. It also may help to prevent fecal stagnation, a factor in colon cancer, appendicitis and IBD. It can be used as a non-invasive treatment for hemorrhoids too.

# 3. INDIVIDUAL DIET – FIND THE LEAST HARMING FOOD FOR YOU

Hippocrates' wisdom has not vanished anywhere. Real food, without additives can still heal you.

The idea is to find healing foods that do not have any, or foods that have very limited allergic reactions and possible harm to your body.

It will take time to discover what they are, but there are foods that suit you too! Because we are all individuals, it is impossible to say exactly what suits your specific gut. However, there are many empty foods that do not give health benefits and should be avoided as much as possible, for instance excess sugar, flour, chemical salt. Also avoiding gluten and milk is helping many people. On your path to recovery think about the big picture, do not judge yourself too harshly if you fail sometimes.

Today there are many well known diets for gastrointestinal problems to follow such as SCD[tm] (Specific Carbohydrate Diet). As the name implies, you should limit the consumption of unhealthy carbohydrates.

The first thing that I thought when I started following SCD[tm] was "does my cooking really have to be this complicated?". I soon learned that I was eating much simpler foods and they made me feel better.

No matter what diet you follow, if it's Paleo, a whole food plant-based diet, Vegetarian, FodMap, a Lectin Avoidance Diet, bear in mind that you most likely need to combine them if one diet does not work 100%. It is also good to do it with the support of a professional nutritionist.

## ABOUT SCD[TM]

In SCD[tm], there are NO starches, grains, pasta, breads, complex sugars or processed factory-made food, these recipes are actually the base of many healthy diets. Once you realise this and put it into practice, you are on the way to a better gut health!

In the SCD™ diet, the main foods consists of what humans used to eat before agriculture began. It is also `biologically` correct because it is species appropriate. The diet is all organic and real food.

Here are two good studies that prove diet matters tremendously in gastrointestinal problems:

1. A study made in 2015 by Rush University shows SCD™ is effective in healing IBD and it is the largest of its kind. This was a very promising note from the study: "The health a subgroup of patients with IBD has notably improved as a result of following the SCD™." The article was published in the Journal of the Academy of Nutrition and Dietetics. For more information, please check out Elaine Gottschall's book called "Breaking the Vicious Cycle" for the whole SCD™-diet.

2. Can diet alone be used to treat Crohn's disease and Ulcerative Colitis? It is a question Children's Doctor David Suskind, a gastroenterologist in Seattle, has been researching for years and today he finally has the answer: Yes indeed it can!

In a first-of-its-kind-study led by Suskind, published December 2016 in the journal of Clinical Gastroenterology, diet alone was shown to bring pediatric patients with active Crohn's and UC into clinical remission.

## OUR SCD™ EXPERIENCE

My wife has been a lifesaver for me by helping with SCD™ or other specific food preparations. SCD™ can be quite a challenging diet, when you have the normal daily routines to follow or if you simply are too sick to make them. You can't just go to a shop and buy ready-made `SCD™ foods`. So do not feel bad if it is too much to handle when trying to cook all those special meals. Be patient and accept all the help you can get!

There may not be "the one diet that fixes" you totally, but there are great ones that can really help. As I have been tailoring my own diet to fit my life, it is quite obvious that it makes no sense for me to follow the official food pyramid. If I do so, I am back in the hospital in 2–4 weeks. I have made that mistake too many times!

SCD<sup>tm</sup> was my lifeline during the hardest years between 2004–2006, especially the SCD<sup>tm</sup> 24hr yogurt helped me to build a better microbioma in my gut. Homemade yogurt is one of the best foods that greatly improve the amount of beneficial bacteria:

1. One cup (236ml) has about 708 billion beneficial bacteria (breakingtheviciouscycle.info)
2. Total Viable Bacteria – a commercial product has also a great amount, 83 billion CFUs. (tested by Labdoor, an independent company that tests food supplements)

Diet may not be the only cause of IBD, but it sure has a big role in it! Certain foods may trigger a flare-up or make symptoms worse. Those triggers can vary widely from person to person and no one type of food or beverage aggravates symptoms for all people with IBD. Many people I have met have one thing in common – grains and starches (lectin) make them sick.

Another thing that relieves symptoms is eating berries daily. They are plants that contain polyphenols. Meaning that polyphenol-rich foods are super-nutritious, they even have anticancer agents and are used as potential chemotherapeutic food. Pomegranate is another great example.

By eating polyphenol rich food, you are getting the most nutrients from your food!

So, if you have access to them, you should add them to your daily diet.

Polyphenols:
• help digestion
• decrease inflammation
• boost immune system
• lower the risk of heart disease (No 1 killer in USA)
• balance cholesterol

The richest sources of polyphenols are various spices and dried herbs, cocoa products, some dark coloured berries, some seeds (flaxseed) and nuts (chestnut, hazelnut) and some vegetables, including olive and globe artichoke heads. Aronia, pomegranate, mulberry, bitter melon and green tea are also good choices as polyphenol sources.

**Top 10 polyphenol-rich foods**

- Cloves
- Star anise
- Cocoa powder
- Mexican oregano, dried
- Celery seed
- Black chokeberry
- Dark chocolate
- Flaxseed meal
- Black elderberry
- Chestnut

# AVOIDING HARMFUL FOODS

For people with extreme symptoms, the simplest way to identify "- the right trigger foods" is to first follow an elimination diet for a minimum of 5 to 7 days. If you want to be sure, 23 days is better — following a meal plan that avoids all potential offending foods, then slowly reintroducing the same foods one by one. Another easier way is to check the allergens using blood tests and a proper medicine center. The downside is that not everyone can afford it. The procedure can easily cost over 1000 $ / 950 €. Some symptoms can appear after few days after eating, so how can you tell exactly where they came from unless you are using the blood test? I think it is well worth it. After the test, you may be surprised to discover that you did not know that those ingredients could trigger and/or keep the inflammation in your gut!

In the last hundred years, the increase in many different artificial sweeteners, chemical additives and pesticides in the diet has led us to a never been seen before problematic situation. We are creating new health problems all the time.

We are seeing more obesity than ever and also more absorption problems that lead to weight loss and malnutrition conditions. Our bodies have not adapted to absorb the chemicals well because they are unnatural and we most likely will never do so. Therefore we should take a closer look at what we ate 10,000–15,000 years ago, as being the food our human race should consume because our digestion can only be adapted over time.

* Elimination diet

Why should you follow this type of diet? Well, to eliminate the harmful ingredients from your diet that may trigger your inflammation. You can also do this without any pre-test and find out the allergens by yourself, but it is much more difficult and time consuming.

**Avoid these for 23 days:**
No gluten, sugar, dairy, eggs, peanuts, corn, soy, fast food or alcohol.
Avoid all packaged, processed or fast foods.

Doctor Borok's elimination diet tests with 5000 IBS/IBD people is encouraging.

Dr. G. Borok, a general practitioner in South Africa, has had considerable success with intestinal problems using an elimination and rotation diet developed by Dr. Marshall of Norwalk, Connecticut. In more than 5,000 patients with irritable bowel syndrome (IBS), 99.9% have experienced relief of all bowel symptoms.

"In cases of ulcerative colitis (UC) and Crohn's disease (CD) (IBD), the response rate is between 85% to 90%. Other symptoms, such as those affecting muscles, joints, lungs, and kidneys, as well as emotional symptoms such as depression and anxiety, improve in the 80% to 90% range." - Based on information in: Townsend Letter for Doctors & Patients, April 1998

WHY 23 DAYS?

If you want to be sure, it takes 23 days. Antibodies, which are the proteins that your immune system makes when it reacts to foods, live for around 21 to 23 days before they disappear, so if you do not cut things to which you are sensitive for at least that period of time, then you will not get the full benefit of eliminating them.

## 8 FOODS, THAT ACCOUNT FOR ABOUT 90% OF ALL FOOD-ALLERGY REACTIONS:

| | | | |
|---|---|---|---|
| 1. Milk | 3. Peanuts | 5. Wheat/Gluten | 7. Fish |
| 2. Eggs | 4. Nuts | 6. Soy | 8. Shellfish |

| ELIMINATE | ALTERNATIVE (DURING PERIOD OF ELIMINATION) |
|---|---|
| Gluten | Bone broth |
| Dairy | Raw milk |
| Soy | Fermented foods and probiotics! |
| Corn | Cruciferous vegetables * and leafy greens |
| Peanuts | Coconut products |
| Citrus fruits | Quality proteins (chlorella, nettle, quinoa, sprouted wild rice etc.) |
| Hydrogenated oils / trans fats (fast food, processed foods) | Fats (olive oil, avocado oil, coconut oil, ghee, butter etc.) |
| Sugar | Fresh fruits (very little) |
| Alcohol and caffeine (tea tree has caffeine) | Caffeine free (Rooibos tea etc.) |

* Cruciferous vegetables: Arugula, Bok choi, Broccoli, Brussels sprouts, Cabbage, Cauliflower, Collard greens, Horseradish, Kale, Radishes, Rutabaga, Turnips, Watercress and Wasabi.

After the elimination diet, start enjoying healing foods in your diet.
Start by introducing 1–2 foods at a time for about 5 days to avoid setbacks.

## SUPERFOODS ARE GREAT, BUT USE THESE WITH CAUTION:

1. **Soy-products** (gut problems, immune system problems, cognitive decline, weight gain). Especially men, if you want your sex drive to last, try avoiding soy products. They can cause hormonal imbalance.
2. **Wheatgrass.** High in chlorophyll, but some people have difficulties in digesting grass. Start with a small portion of wheatgrass to see if it agrees with you.
3. **Goji-berries.** They contain lectins, which may disrupt your immune system and prevent your body from healing. Lectins can cause leaky gut and inflammation.

# DIFFERENT MEAL IDEAS

This is not a cook book, so these recipes are just examples of what I and many others have found beneficial. It totally depends on how serious the stage your illness is and what suits your body. The simpler the food is, the better it is to find the right diet for your specific need. If you are on FODMAP or SCD™, use their recipes instead.

## BREAKFAST

1. Fermented yoghurt + berries and honey

2. Raw eggs (organic), rice- or almond milk or similar plus a pinch of raw cane sugar. You can add some cream (organic, no carrageenan food additives) and a drop of olive oil to bring more energy. Later on you can add some raw cocoa, if your stomach can tolerate it. It gives you extra energy!

3. Lightly cooked eggs go well with hard cheese, pepper and sea salt.

4. Quinoa porridge, salt and little honey with some good cheese (the harder the better i.e. parmesan)

5. Buckwheat, millet porridge. To gain weight, rice porridge with cream. Some people can tolerate gluten-free oatmeal.

6. Vegetable soups with carrots, broccoli, cucumber, sweet potatoes, white beans, beet greens, soybeans, lima beans, spinach, lentils and kidney beans. Use microwave as little as possible to keep all the nutrients intact.

7. Smoothies (my favorite) have endless choices! Start with water. Add some avocado, banana, lots of your favorite berries, and a dollop of honey. Combine it with nuts and seeds. Note: Nuts and seeds cause allergic reaction to many. To get more energy from the smoothie, add a spoonful of oil (olive oil, coconut oil etc.).

8. Raw porridge is so easy! Mix gluten free oatmeal and coconut milk (no carrageenan). Add some chia seeds and blueberries/strawberries. Let it soak in the fridge for an hour or overnight. Enjoy!

Especially for work, use a thermos jug. You can put vegetable soup in the jug and enjoy a meal many times during the day. If you really want to have a healthier lunch at work, it can be made with little imagination and your health will flourish.

1. Cooked or steamed vegetables, with some rice and fish. Vegetarian meals are in general gentler on your digestion than meat. Use lentils, different vegetables – the more the merrier – colors represent life and vitality (antioxidants).

2. Vegetable soup – use your preferred vegetables, lentils work beautifully too. Cook them together in water, season with sea salt and pepper, add any other spices you love, along with the herbs you like, and enjoy. You can add coconut cream to make it tastier and richer. If you don't like the taste of coconut, use a bit of organic cream or creme fraiche. If you prefer, puree the soup, it will have a lovely velvety texture and taste to it.

3. Omelette – use organic eggs, beat them and mix with any healthy and tasty ingredient, for example: organic onions, tomatoes, peppers, beans, and a little bit of cheese to your liking, add some sea salt and pepper, and lightly cook in olive oil or real butter using a moderate heat, stirring occasionally. Add some fresh parsley to serve and enjoy. Fresh basil also works well - or any herb you like. Tastes delicious even cold.

4. Wild salmon (hopefully you can find a wild and freely grown fish) - poached, cooked or baked in the oven, but do not overcook. Season with lemon, sea salt, pepper, fresh dill and chives. Serve with cooked or steamed vegetables, and whole grain rice. Healthy and delicious, wild salmon is loaded with omega-3 fatty acids.

5. Make a Greek salad. In a bowl, toss together some fresh tomatoes, chunks of cucumber bits, sliced mild red onions, green peppers and black olives to the plate, mix. Add a thick slice of feta cheese on top. Drizzle some extra virgin olive oil and quality vinegar and finish with some chopped oregano and then enjoy!

6.  Mexican Salad (with or without meat): Mix together some different salad leaves as the bottom layer. Cook some red onion and beans, or alternatively some chicken (organic) files with red onion, as well as yellow, green and red peppers. Season with chilli (which is good for digestion, but not good when the intestines are inflamed), black pepper, sea salt and any (organic) herbs and Mexican spices. Avoid commercial sauces, they are usually filled with preservatives, artificial flavors and colorings.

7.  Asparagus – pick a fresh and firm bunch of asparagus. Cook the asparagus in water with a pinch of sea salt and coconut sugar. Cook for about 7 minutes ("-al dente", no overcooking). Place them on a plate, side by side, about 4–5 stalks per person. Mash one hard-boiled organic egg, per person, and sprinkle on top of the asparagus with some melted organic butter. Finish with ground black pepper and top with shredded parmesan. Voila!

## DESSERTS AND SNACKS

### Banana pancakes

1 organic banana
2 organic eggs
Pinch of ceylon cinnamon
Pinch of cardamon

Mix all ingredients together to form a batter. Then fry a small ladleful of the mix in a shallow pan of coconut oil to form a pancake over a gentle heat. Sprinkle shredded coconut on top along with your favourite berries. Healthy, simple, gluten free and delicious!

### Kale chips

Place some kale leaves on a baking tray. Add some quality salt, sprinkle a little olive oil on top and heat in the oven (350° F / 175° C) for 10–15 minutes.

There are plenty of healthy and delicious `raw´ cakes, so if your stomach can tolerate them, enter this gluten-free world and forget the old fashioned flour cakes.

# GUT SPECIFIC FOODS AND RECIPES

About conversions:
1 T. (tablespoons) = 3 tsp. (teaspoons)
4 cups = 1 quart = 0,95 Litres

Probiotic Foods with Good Bacteria for Your Gut: SCD™-yogurt, kombucha, sauerkraut, pickles, miso, tempeh, natto, kimchi, raw cheese (goat, sheep, A2 cows soft cheeses). Organic probiotic yogurt from goat or sheep milk.

## LINSEED GEL

1 cup of linseeds (20 ml)
4 cups of water (1 L)
1 cup (20 ml) of turmeric + some ground black pepper (pepper/piperine will boost the turmeric's power)

This gel will help you to renew and strengthen the bacteria and boost immunity.

**Instructions:**
- Boil the water and linseeds.
- Keep it on a low temperature with the lid on for 10 minutes. Check and add water if needed.
- Add turmeric and a hint of black pepper and let it stand for another 10 minutes.
- Strain the gel into another pan and throw away the linseeds. I did the opposite the first time by accident, that's why I explain it here :-)
- When the gel has cooled down, keep it refrigerated.
- Drink ½ cup at once. Drink it warm if possible (not hot, boiling water harms the gentle ingredients).
- Regimen: 1st week: 3 x / day  2nd week: 2 x / day  3rd week: 1 x / day

Kefir, kombucha or some other beverage that are live probiotic drinks will help you to get the good bacteria we all need.

## COCO – GINGER ANTI-INFLAMMATORY DRINK

(for all kinds of inflammations in the body)

4–5 tablespoons of coconut oil
1 inch piece of ginger root
Turmeric
2 cups of coconut milk / almond milk (50 ml)
Some cinnamon and cardamom
Honey

**Instructions:**
- Grate the ginger (works best if it is fresh) and turmeric (or use a powder), heat the coconut oil in a very mild temperature (90°F/33°C) for 2–4 minutes only.
- Add coconut- or almond milk and mix them well.
- Add the spices (cinnamon and cardamom)
- Sweeten with organic honey. It is most beneficial if enjoyed warm (not hot).
- Recipe is from a Baltic healer and Leena Nicolaou (Finland/Cyprus)

## RAW – ANTI - INFLAMMATORY DRINK

2 tsp. raw and organic apple cider vinegar
1 tsp. turmeric powder (or squeeze turmeric into liquid)
Hint of a black pepper (to improve the bioavailability of turmeric)
1/2 lemon (juice)
1/2 tsp. cayenne pepper
1 tsp. honey
1/2 cup of water (10-20 ml)

(Markku Saarinen powershot)

## BONE BROTH

Good for immune system, gut, joints and bones. It may even overcome food intolerances and allergies.

**Ingredients:**
- organic bones, game or beef
- 2 table spoons of organic apple cider vinegar
- water

Fill a large pot with water, add the bones, vinegar and these ingredients:
- bit of ginger
- onion, carrot, celery, garlic
- fresh herbs, such as thyme, parsley and/or rosemary
- 2 bay leaves
- 1 teaspoonful sesameseed oil or coconut oil and some seasalt.

Cook the bones for a long time, from 8 hours up to 24 hours – the longer the better.

Once ready, put it in an airtight container in the refrigerator for 4–6 hours or overnight. This will allow the fat to rise to the top and solidify. Scrape the fat off the top with a spoon. This will leave you with a gelatinous bone broth when cold. It will be good to eat for several weeks.

**Tip:** freeze the broth in ice cube molds and use whenever you like.

## ANTI-INFLAMMATORY FOOD INGREDIENTS:

Bone broth, celery, beet, black beans, bok choy (chinese cabbage), broccoli, red peppers, salmon, flaxseed, tomato, coconut oil and of course ginger and turmeric. Also clove, rosemary, cinnamon, jamaican allspice, apple pie spice mixture, oregano, pumpkin pie spice mixture, marjoram, sage, thyme.

## NATURAL ANTIBIOTICS:

Apple cider vinegar (organic!), ginger, horseradish root, onion, habanero peppers, oregano oil, turmeric, echinacea herb, raw honey, garlic.

## ANTI-INFLAMMATORY SMOOTHIE INGREDIENTS

Apple, avocado, apricot, banana, berries, cherries, pineapple, cantaloupe, grapes, kiwi, orange, papaya, pineapple, carrot, green leafy vegetables, celery, spinach. Almonds, walnuts, and macadamia nuts. Extra virgin olive oil, coconut oil, chia seeds (let them soak 20 min before consuming), hemp powder, cocoa, ginger and turmeric. Use pure water or green tea.

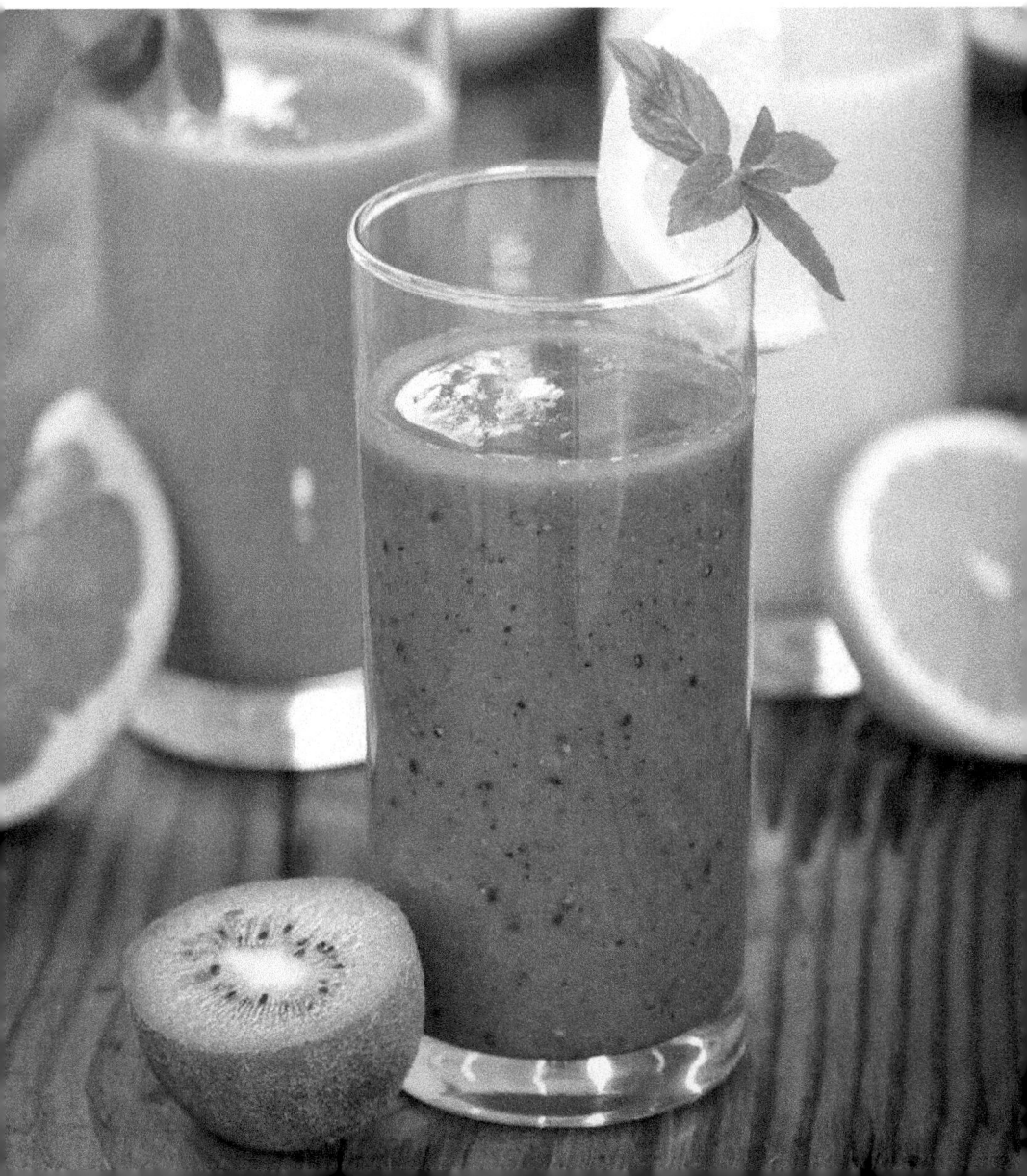

# HEALTHY OILS

Add 1–2 tablespoons of extra virgin olive oil to your daily diet, 3 times a day to make it even healthier. To make it taste better I use some organic apple juice. Remember to add enough oils to your diet, also to add fish oil after the elimination diet. Your brain needs this too!

Olive oil – The corner stone of Mediterranean diet

Consumption of olive oil per capita in Greece compared to other countries 2011–2012:
- Greece 39 lb (17,9 kg)
- England 1 lb (0,9 kg)
- USA 2 lb (1,1 kg)
- Australia 4 lb (2,1 kg)

The figures have been highest in countries that are situated in the Southern Mediterranean such as Portugal, Cyprus, Italy and Spain 247 – 444 oz (7-12,6 kg). Also Morocco and Tunis are big consumers. Olive oil definitely has a role in a healthy diet, which is why the Mediterranean diet (vegetables, beans, fish and fruits etc.) is known as one of the healthiest in the planet.

Greeks also need to consume lots of olive oil for antioxidant protection. Greece has among the most smokers in the world (51.7% of adults smoke; on average 16 cigarettes per smoker per day).

## THE HEAVY PRICE OF GLOBALIZATION IS SEEN AROUND THE GLOBE

The globalization is affecting very fast also in the Mediterranean area. As of today (2018) many Greeks are forced to move away from the villages in to the big cities, which often means forgetting the traditional, healthy food. Regional/country data (WHO, 2016) informs that boys in Greece had the highest obesity rates in Europe, 16.7% of the population respectively.

Children and adolescents have rapidly transitioned from mostly underweight to mostly overweight in many middle-income countries, including in East Asia, Latin America and the Caribbean. A study by Imperial College London and WHO predicts that world will have more obese children and adolescents than underweight by 2022.

No matter how healthy the oil is; coconut oil, olive oil, peanut oil, red palm oil, avocado oil etc. Always use unrefined and cold pressed oils. Please make sure your product is made under sustainable agriculture, that is the way to show to Mother Earth some TLC. Rotating oils is a great idea as it gives the body the different combo of essential fatty acids which it needs. Butter is pure natural dairy product and margarine highly processed product made from vegetable oil.

Protect all sensitive oils with care:
- Keep them in a cool, dark place
- Use smaller bottles rather than larger ones to ensure freshness
- Replace the cap immediately after each use
- To prevent from oxidation, use a drop of lemon juice or astaxanthin in the oil

WANT TO SEE OXIDATION IN ACTION? SLICE AN APPLE AND PUT LEMON OIL (OR ORANGE OIL) ON ONE HALF AND LEAVE THE OTHER HALF WITHOUT IT. YOU'LL SEE HOW THE ANTIOXIDANTS (VITAMIN C) PROTECT THE APPLE FROM OXIDATION AND TURNING BROWN. THIS IS THE SAME WAY YOU SHOULD THINK ABOUT YOUR CELLS. PREVENT THEM FROM OXIDATION!

Consider avoiding these oils:
- Soybean oil
- Corn oil
- Cottonseed oil
- Canola oil
- Sunflower oil

Cooking with vegetable oils such as corn oil or sunflower oil releases toxic chemicals linked to cancer and other diseases, scientists are now recommending food be fried in olive oil, coconut oil, butter or even lard.

**Is taking palm oil new to you?**

In 2013, the journal BMC Complementary and Alternative Medicine published a study that evaluated the antioxidant activity of oil palm leaf extract (OPLE) in mice that had diabetes, which was given orally. They noticed that oxidative stress markers and inflammation, which are directly related to the most common causes of death in the world (cancer and heart disease) began to decrease. Palm oil also has more vitamin A and E than any other plant based oil. However, there are serious environmental concerns related to the rapid increase in palm oil production. Make sure you only choose companies that are committed to sustainable palm oil.

# HEALTHY DRINKS

1. APPLE CIDER VINEGAR: **2 tsp. of apple cider vinegar (organic and unfiltered) with 1 cup of water. Apple cider vinegar contains important enzymes and friendly bacteria for better intestine and overall health. Highly recommended and is a healthy way to start the day :)**

2. COFFEE AND WATER: **Drink 2 glasses of water with every cup of organic coffee. The diuretic effect of caffeine increases your urine output. By drinking water you can lessen the dehydration effect that coffee creates. The water you consume each day is more important than any other nutrient in your diet. When your stomach is upset, leaving coffee out may help your symptoms.**

3. ORGANIC RAW CANE SUGAR + SALT: **One spoonful of raw cane sugar with 1/4 tsp himalayan salt (or similar). Use salt that still has minerals in it. All salts are not equal, in terms of their impact on your health. Prefer unprocessed natural salt, it has many essential biological functions. Minimize the use of processed table salt.**

4. LEMON AND WATER: **Good for liver, cleanses the blood and boosts pH-levels. Remember that all citrus fruits contain acids that can damage your teeth enamel. Enamel is hard to grow back and once it's severely damaged, it can even be irreparable.**

Try cold lemon water instead of warm lemon water. This will reduce the amount of available acid that can touch your teeth. Here are some tips to lessen the damages:
• Try lemon essential oil instead. It has all the benefits, but the oil is made from the lemon peel, not the fruit which is why it's better for your teeth! 1–2 drops in a glass of water is enough.
• Use a straw to bypass the teeth.
• Rinse your mouth with water before brushing your teeth. When citric acid is still fresh, it will wear away the enamel.

5. WATER: (lukewarm), turmeric and ground pepper (piperine, the key chemical in black pepper is required to multiply the power of turmeric). Add some ginger and honey which results in more resistance and a stronger immune system. Excellent way to get rid of the flu too!

6. COCONUT MILK: (sugarfree and from a metal free can) with 1 tablespoon of chia seeds (let the seeds soak for at least 20 minutes or leave them in the fridge over night). Great source of Omega-3 fatty acids.

Also Kombucha, aloe vera, camu, noni, blueberry, pomegranate, vegetable juices, kvass (raw and unpasteurized), and fermented teas are all great choices.

# SUPPLEMENTS

The following supplements have been beneficial to me over the years. You can think about taking some of them to your daily regimen, but remember to switch them every now and then. Talk with a nutritionist to find out about the right quantity of supplements to take and when it is best to take them. If it says 1 tablet daily, you may need 5–10 times more to get the 'therapeutic' dosage. Please remember that higher dosages need to be controlled and not taken over a long period of time. Avoid synthetic vitamins and supplements if possible.

1. PROBIOTICS for healthy gut biota. Probiotic yeast, boulardii can reach the gut alive. It should contain at least these three common good bacterias that encourage healthy digestion and maintain levels of immunity:

- L. acidophilus
- B. Longum
- B. bifidum (found in both the small and large intestine)

However, the truth is that we or should I say the scientific community don't know yet if more bacteria are actually better for us or how many different strains of probiotic bacteria are in the gut to begin with. What we do know is that they are vital to our well being.

## 2. GLUTAMINE

Glutamine, occasionally even 10g daily. Infected intestines can not produce enough of it. It speeds up the healing of the infection. It rarely causes problems, but for long term use also take B vitamins, especially vitamin B12, which controls glutamine build up in the body. It is very beneficial to the whole body, not just to gut health.

- improves gastrointestinal health
- heals ulcers and leaky gut, IBS and reduces diarrea
- helps memory and concentration
- cuts cravings (alcohol and sweets)
- treats diabetes and blood sugar
- improves muscle growth

## 3. ENZYMES

Digestive enzymes aid digestion by breaking down the foods into nutrients and waste. If proper digestion doesn't take place, we experience gastrointestinal discomfort along with nutrient deficiencies. Why do some people prefer eating raw foods? If you can eat your food raw, you'll get the most nutrition from your food in its natural state. The best temperature for enzymes is body temperature, so cooking and processing food destroys them.

## 4. VITAMIN C (EVEN 1000 MG, 4 X A DAY FOR 2-4 WEEKS)

- boosts the immune system
- heals wounds
- enables health promotion and disease prevention
- combats oxidative damage

- reduces cellular DNA damage (first step in cancer initiation)
- speeds up the healing and recovery processes.

## 5. MULTIVITAMIN

- Liquid and vegetable-based multivitamins are absorbed better

## 6. IRON

- Iron is a mineral responsible for carrying oxygen in your red blood cells and transmitting nerve impulses.
- Iron deficiency may occur when feeling dizzy, weak, tired, having headaches or looking pale
- Iron deficiency occurs in about 60-80% of patients with inflammatory bowel disease (IBD). Check ferritin levels regularly with blood test.

## 7. VITAMIN-B12

- Energy levels
- Red blood cells
- DNA and nervous system

B12 is important especially to
- Those who have had surgery in the last part of the small intestine (B12 absorbs there).
- Vegans
- Elderly people

## 8. OMEGA-3

Omega-3 has anti-inflammatory and Omega-6 has pro-inflammatory benefits.

Why do we need Omega-6 then? Inflammation helps protect our bodies from infection and injury. But when the inflammatory response is inappropriate or excessive, it can cause severe damage and it can contribute to disease. Overly excessive inflammation may be one of the leading causes of the most serious diseases that we are dealing with today, including IBS, heart disease, metabolic syndrome, diabetes, arthritis, Alzheimer's, many types of cancer, etc.

If you are in doubt of the Omega-3 and Omega-6 ratio, take a blood test. The ratio should be close to 1:1. If you eat a typical western diet, the ratio can be as high as 1:20.

Omega chart. Watch out for an overconsumption of Omegas with products that are high in Omega-6s.

| OIL | OMEGA-3 % | OMEGA-6 % |
|-----|-----------|-----------|
| Fish | 100 | 0 |
| Flaxseed | 57 | 14 |
| Walnut | 10 | 52 |
| Soybean | 7 | 51 |
| Sunflower | 0 | 65 |
| Corn | 0 | 54 |

NOTE! You can take both olive oil and omega-3 together and have all the benefits.

## 9. VITAMIN-D

Vitamin D is one of the most important micronutrients. Nearly every tissue and cell in our body has a vitamin D receptor.

• Important for good overall health
• It fights against disease
• Boosts immune system
• Reduces depression
• It belongs to fat soluble vitamins group (A,D,E,K)

Check the status of your vitamin D levels through blood tests. 100 to 150 nmol/L is ideal.

About Vitamin D toxicity: If you take 40,000 IU / 1000 μg per day for a couple of months or longer, or take a very large one time dose, 300,000 IU / 7500 μg you may get an overdose (hypercalcemia).

While sun products help to protect against skin cancer – they also block a majority of your body's vitamin D production (even 97%), so being in the sun doesn't always give enough vitamin D.

## 10. MELATONIN

- Take it just before bedtime
- Regarding anti-inflammatory and antioxidant abilities, melatonin has been found beneficial in several experimental and clinical studies including IBD. Inflammation and oxidative process are associated with IBD.
- Strengthens the immune system

## 11. OTHER

### Cannabis
Many people who suffer from inflammatory bowel disease (IBD) are turning to cannabis (or medical marijuana) to ease some of the symptoms of the disease. Today (2018) there are 29 legal medical marijuana states in USA alone. To avoid misunderstanding we need to establish the specific cannabinoids, as well as appropriate medical conditions, optimal dose, and mode of administration, to maximize the beneficial effects while avoiding any potential harmful effects of cannabinoid use.

### Other beneficial supplements
- MSM (with vitamin-C), helps to heal wounded tissues. After the gym helps the muscles to recover.
- Essential oils like tea tree, frankincense and peppermint. Use 100% pure essential oils.
- Coptis root. This is great for diarrea and acute inflammation. It has a strong antibacterial effect on staphylococcus, streptococcus, pneumococcus, but poor antibacterial effect on E. coli, Proteus, and Salmonella typhi.

Did I miss something? I am sure I did! There are numerous traditional ways from Chinese medicine to Ayurveda. Explore the world to find the healing herbs your body needs!

# ANOTHER APPROACH BY FUNCTIONAL MEDICINE

The medical system we live in today allows doctors to treat you mainly using their acute care approach to medicine. Also the fact that doctors often do not have enough time to solve the patients real problems forces them to quickly write prescription drugs. Chemicals do not save us, if we have not seen that yet, very soon we will. There is no doubt that we still need drugs or surgery, but we also need a different approach, with methodology and tools that are specifically designed to prevent gently all diseases. Functional Medicine is a much more 'wholistic' and may be the evolution in the practice of medicine that better addresses the healthcare needs of the 21st century. If you are not getting answers from your doctor, maybe it's time to turn to functional medicine.

THE NEW AND FUTURISTIC APPROACH TO HEALTHCARE IS PERSONALIZED MEDICINE TO ADDRESS OUR INDIVIDUAL GENETICS.

# OIC - OH I SEE IT NOW

I have now entered a stage in my life that I
am being guided by something greater than
I can comprehend. My true belief is that the
very best effort we can make for living a
happy and healthy life is to stop the causes
that make us sick. A healthy diet, a loving
family, love towards life, gratitude, enough
rest and exercise and a peaceful mind are a
huge part of the whole.

Tommi Sundqvist

"IF I CAN PLANT
EVEN A SMALL
SEED OF HOPE
FOR SOMEONE,
THIS HAS BEEN
WORTH IT."

# PASI HEINONEN & SANNA KOSTAMO

Both want to share their stories too.
I truly thank them from the bottom of my
heart and let them also give you hope.
They both are great examples of
motivation and determination to achieve
the best health and quality of life.
Well done!

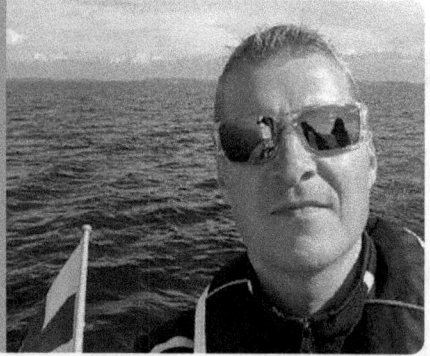

PASI HEINONEN (46)

ENTREPRENEUR
TURKU
FINLAND

I was diagnosed with very aggressive Ulcerative Colitis in my colon in 2005. The doctor's first comment after the medical examination and during diagnosis was "with medicine you can cope with this, but you will have to take prescription medicine for the rest of your life." For nine years my Colitis was manageable and life was normal. Then in 2014, my colitis became so bad that cortisone was added (60mg a day) on top of my normal medicine (Asacol x 5, 800mg). It calmed down for a few months. During the fall of 2015, my Colitis flared up again and cortisone was added, again. The same thing happened, it calmed down for a few months. At the end of the year I had to start using cortisone for the third time. But it didn´t work as before, the inflammation had started to increase even before the medicine period was over. I knew something else had to be done. The medicine was simply not working anymore.

That was when I decided to get help by changing my diet. February 2016 was the biggest turning point in my life. I also contacted Tommi after my wife saw his presentation about IBD. Even though changing my eating habits was a big step and it had taken lots of research, new thinking and determination, it was worth it 100%. My family fully supported me and my dear wife had already been eating healthily, which all helped me a lot.

Already after a few weeks, I started to feel positive changes in my gut. After three months all my symptoms were gone. After four months I took Cal pro inflammation tests and they were as low as a healthy person's values. My Cal pro had decreased from 783 to 73 and down to 18 in one year (2015–2016).

The same year I did my own microbiome tests, and importantly an allergy test for 280 foods which helped me find the foods that may trigger allergy and inflammation. I decided to stop using Asacol in November 2016 and to follow a healthy diet with supplements.

I have now been without medicine for four months and I feel really good. I am fully aware that I may suffer from violent episodes in the future, but the experiences in Spring 2016 were so positive that I am confident that the path is right for me now. I have a good feeling that I can manage Colitis without medicine. On top of that I don't have to worry about the side effects of the pharmaceutical drugs. Thumbs up!

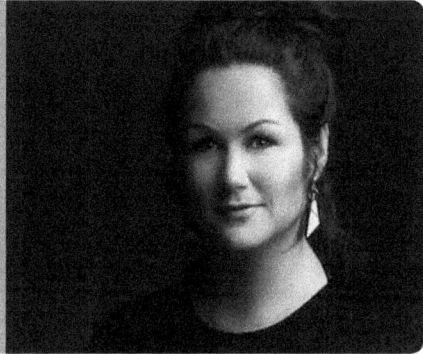

SANNA KOSTAMO (38)

ENTREPRENEUR
PHOTOGRAPHER
CREATIVE DESIGNER
JYVÄSKYLÄ, FINLAND

This is my story of Crohn's disease and how I have dealt with it. My first symptoms started when I was 29 years old, after my trip to Istanbul in 2008. I had severe stomach cramps, high rates of infection, diarrhea and fever, which had started re-occuring every 6 months.

I was finally diagnosed with Crohn's disease in 2012. When I got home from the hospital, I watched a TV programme, with Dr. Olli Sovijärvi explaining the importance of diet and healthy living, in treating autoimmune diseases. Olli Sovijärvi is a Licensed General Practitioner at Helsinki Antioxidant Clinic. He is one of the pioneers in holistic medicine in Finland. The program hit me hard, so I started to explore the topic. I started following the Paleo diet, but discovered it was not suitable for me on the whole. I picked up many good things from the diet though, such as using natural and unprocessed food, avoiding grain, dairy products and sugars.

Due to the recommendation of another doctor I started taking Pentasa medication. Despite taking it my Crohn's continued to flare up every six months or so. My Cal pro levels were 3000–4000 at the highest. Finally I started having long periods of fever, the reason for this was never discovered despite of numerous tests. I therefore decided to stop taking the Pentasa medication, and my fevers stopped.

I was told to eat Cortison and Azamun to calm down the Crohn's. I did not give up, even when I started to feel desperate. I eventually started getting pain in my back and hips. I realised that I had to make a greater change, so I stayed away from my stressful job, to continue my studies in photography, which is one of my dream jobs. My Cal pro values were 800 at this point, so my intestines were not functioning well. After taking time off from work, things started improving for me.

I finally had an appointment with Dr. Olli Sovijärvi, and at the same time Tommi Sundqvist contacted me, to help him with his book. I was happy to help. More people had started to appear in my life, supporting me in my healing process. I felt I was on the right path. At the antioxidant clinic Dr. Sovijärvi had my intestines analyzed as well as having allergy bloodtest, to check out 85 different food substances. The analysis reported that I had very little `good` bacteria and a lot of bad bacteria. Also there were food substances that I was allergic to, without even knowing it, such as egg that I had always consumed a lot. Also my levels of fatty acids were checked. I had too much Omega 6, and too little Omega 3. Dr. Sovijärvi guided me to acupuncture. He advised me on my diet and food supplements, as well as having to do breathing exercises and reminded of the importance of a good sleep. As a consequence, my Cal pro values started to normalize to 40–70. My Crohn's has not been active since 2015.

Today I am very excited about juicing greens. They are very healthy and they really help the body to heal itself. One dosage of green juice a day is good, but sometimes it is good to have a fast with green juices only. Our diet is lacking so many nutrients today, so green juicing helps tremendously. Today my Crohn's is in full remission and I have no pains whatsoever. I really hope my story can help you by giving you light and hope in your path.

Remember, there is always hope when you make changes that help you. My advice to you is: "Take time to do what makes your soul happy."

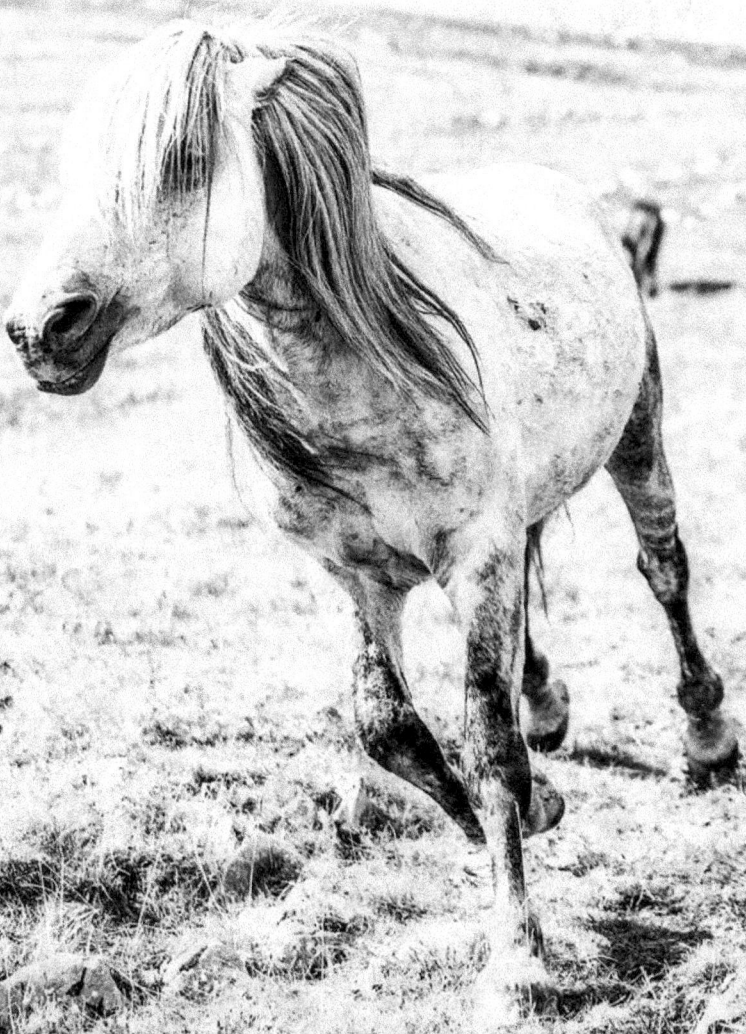

"TAKE TIME TO DO WHAT
MAKES YOUR SOUL HAPPY."

The Universe is my God
Nature is my church
Here I can heal my hurts...

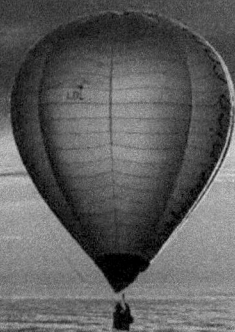

Strong emotional charge is the most important factor for me in photography...

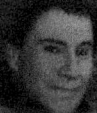

I started my journey of photography as an aerial photographer in Texas. Freedom of flying is still enviting me to get above the clouds into hidden gardens out of our sight. There is so much to experience in pure nature that it's beyond my imagination every time I find my way there.

Marko Airismeri

MA

# YOUR OWN NOTES

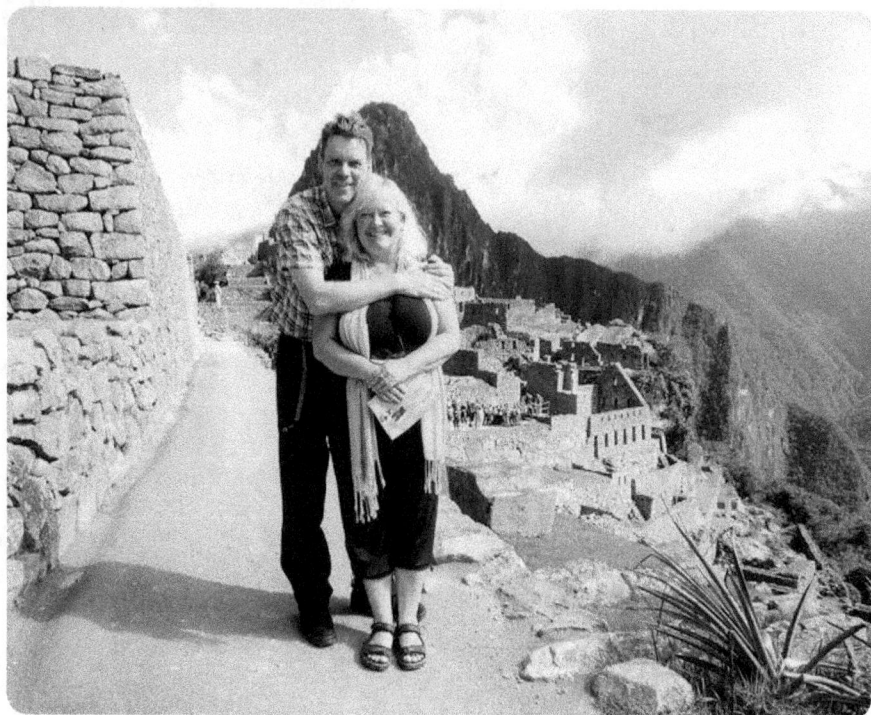

EXPLORE ALL THE
ROADS THAT BRING YOU
VIBRANT HEALTH AND
TRUE HAPPINESS!

THE END

# SOURCES

## GUT BACTERIA IS CRUCIAL IN OUR LIFE

- 7 Benefits of Natural Childbirth, by Lilian Presti (accessed June 1, 2017)
  http://naturallysavvy.com/nest/the-benefits-of-natural-childbirth#sthash.zR4Ja7ik.dpuf
- Vaginal Birth vs. C-Section: Pros & Cons, by Cari Nierenberg, Live Science Contributor (March 20, 2015). http://www.livescience.com/45681-vaginal-birth-vs-c-section.html
- Diet-Induced Dysbiosis of the Intestinal Microbiota and the Effects on Immunity and Disease. Published online 2012 Aug 21. Kirsty Brown,† Daniella DeCoffe,† Erin Molcan, and Deanna L. Gibson* https://www.ncbi.nlm.nih.gov/pmc/articles/PMC3448089/

## DIGESTIVE SYSTEM – IN A NUTSHELL

- American Journal of Roentgenology. 1968;104: 522-524. 10.2214/ajr.104.3.522
  Study: SMALL INTESTINE TRANSIT TIME IN THE NORMAL SMALL BOWEL STUDY, SEUK KY KIM, M.D.
  http://www.ajronline.org/doi/abs/10.2214/ajr.104.3.522
- Study: Human gut microbiota in obesity and after gastric bypass. October 15, 2008. Accessed January 2017. vol. 106 no. 7. Husen Zhang, 2365–2370, doi: 10.1073/pnas.0812600106
  http://www.pnas.org/content/106/7/2365.long
- VIVO - pathophysiology, Gastrointestinal Transit: How long does it take?
  http://www.vivo.colostate.edu/hbooks/pathphys/digestion/basics/transit.html
- The size of the stomach
  http://www.innerbody.com/image/digeov.htm
- Kobra: Animal bytes of the San Diego Zoo)

## IBD – INFLAMMATORY BOWEL DISEASE

- BACKGROUND ABOUT CROHN. Accessed September 2016.
- Use of complementary and alternative medicine in Germany – a survey of patients with inflammatory bowel disease.
- Stefanie Joos12*, Thomas Rosemann1, Joachim Szecsenyi1, Eckhart G Hahn2, Stefan N Willich3 and Benno Brinkhaus23
  biomedcentral.com/1472-6882/6/19/
- International Foundation for Functional Gastrointestinal Disorders, aboutibs.org/pdfs/IBSRealWorld.pdf
- Crohn's and colitis foundation of America, http://www.ccfa.org/resources/surgery-for-crohns-uc.html
- Mayo Clinic, mayoclinic.org/healthy-lifestyle/consumer-health/in-depth/alternative-medicine/art-20045267
- http://worldibdday.org

## LEAKY GUT

- Autoimmunity Reviews. Volume 14, Issue 6, June 2015, Pages 479-489
  http://www.sciencedirect.com/science/article/pii/S1568997215000245
- New research suggests additional evidence that Parkinson's disease may originate in the gut. April 26, 2017 By Maureen Salamon, HealthDay Reporter. (HealthDay News)
  https://consumer.healthday.com/cognitive-health-information-26/parkinson-s-news-526/parkinson-s-disease-may-originate-in-gut-study-says-722060.html

- Jill Carnahan, MD. Leaky Gut – The Syndrome Linked to Many Autoimmune Diseases. July 7, 2014
  http://www.jillcarnahan.com/2014/07/07/leaky-gut-syndrome-linked-many-autoimmune-diseases/
- Pub Med. August 2016, Dietary emulsifiers impact the mouse gut microbiota promoting colitis
  and metabolic syndrome. 2016 Aug 11;536(7615):238. PubMed PMID: 25731162; PubMed Central
  PMCID: PMC4910713. https://www.ncbi.nlm.nih.gov/pubmed/25731162
- Dr. Josh Axe, DNM, DC, CNS. Common Food Additive Promotes Colon Cancer in Mice. April 2017
  https://draxe.com/food-additive-colon-cancer/
- Disabled world. March 2017. http://www.disabled-world.com/artman/publish/leaky-gut.shtml
- Excerpts  from Updated report by The Cornucopia Institute / April 2016.
  Carrageenan - New Studies Reinforce Link to Inflammation, Cancer and Diabetes
- Calprotectin, Alpha laboratories, Accessed january 2017.
  http://www.calprotectin.co.uk/about-calprotectin/
- The International Foundation for Functional Gastrointestinal Disorders (IFFGD).
  http://www.foodsafetynews.com/2016/11/board-nixes-use-of-carrageenan-in-organic-food-
  production/#.WkzJ8zeYPv9
- University of Maryland - Medical Center. Accessed january 2017.
  https://umm.edu/health/medical/altmed/condition/irritable-bowel-syndrome
- Treating IBS and Diarrhea: Diet, Medications, Supplements, and More. Accessed january 2017.
  http://www.webmd.com/ibs/treating-diarrhea
- The colon therapist network. October 2017.
  http://www.colonhealth.net/colon_hydrotherapy/ct_funct.htm
- The International Foundation for Functional Gastrointestinal Disorders (IFFGD).
- University of Maryland - Medical Center
  https://umm.edu/health/medical/altmed/condition/irritable-bowel-syndrome

SCIENCE IS HELPING US TO LIVE HEALTHIER

- https://www.nlm.nih.gov/medlineplus/ency/article/000816.htm
- http://wwf.panda.org/about_our_earth/teacher_resources/webfieldtrips/toxics/our_chemical_world/
- http://articles.mercola.com/sites/articles/archive/2013/12/11/8-flame-retardant-facts.aspx
- https://www.nlm.nih.gov/medlineplus/ency/article/002224.htm
- http://masteringmealtime.com/more-family-time.html
- https://www.foodallergy.org/facts-and-stats
- http://www.calicolabs.com/news/2015/07/21/
- https://www.neb.com

MY STORY

- https://www.sciencedaily.com/releases/2017/05/170529133711.htm
- http://www.healthline.com/health/crohns-disease/ibs-vs-ibd#Overview1

3 WAKE-UP CALLS

- https://www.statnews.com/2017/03/07/alternative-therapies-chart/
- https://www.medicalnewsbulletin.com/new-treatment-for-crohns-disease-mongersen/
- http://wellness.yale.edu/wellness-self-care/community-resources

3. SURGERY -  A BLESSING IN DISGUISE

- (*) Pub Med: http://www.ncbi.nlm.nih.gov/pubmed/15674913

- Department of Paediatric Gastroenterology, Central Manchester and Manchester Children's University Hospitals, Booth Hall Children's Hospital, Charlestown Road, Blackley, Manchester, UK, M9 7AA.

## 2 MAJOR SURGERIES IN 7 DAYS

- https://www.theguardian.com/society/2015/jun/30/bowel-cancer-patients-dying-unnecessarily-care-failure-nhs

## MRSA

- http://www.pharmacytimes.com/contributor/sean-kane-pharmd/2017/03/which-antibiotics-are-most-associated-with-causing-clostridium-difficile-diarrhea

## CAL-PRO - A TEST TO DETECT INFLAMMATION IN THE INTESTINES

- http://articles.mercola.com/sites/articles/archive/2015/12/09/colonoscopy-pros-cons.aspx
- https://www.youtube.com/watch?v=gL3frk2CUYI
- Screening for colorectal cancer: a targeted, updated systematic review for the U.S. Preventive Services Task Force.
- Whitlock EP1, Lin JS, Liles E, Beil TL, Fu R.
- 1 - Kaiser Permanente Center for Health Research, Portland, Oregon, USA.
- https://www.ncbi.nlm.nih.gov/pubmed/28325724
- BMJ Case Rep. 2017 Mar 21;2017. pii: bcr2016219178. doi: 10.1136/bcr-2016-219178.
- Air everywhere: colon perforation after colonoscopy.
- Araújo AV1, Santos C1, Contente H1, Branco C1.
- 1 - Hospital Sao Francisco Xavier, Lisboa, Portugal.

## CLEANING THE INTESTINES GENTLY BEFORE COLONOSCOPY

- https://www.youtube.com/watch?v=gL3frk2CUYI
  "Colon health and the dangers of colonoscopies"
- https://articles.mercola.com/sites/articles/archive/2015/12/09/colonoscopy-pros-cons.aspx

## GOODBYE MEDICINE

- http://www.yourlawyer.com/topics/overview/remicade#sthash.aoO2FJcQ.dpuf
- http://www.breakingtheviciouscycle.info/

## DOCTORS HAVE BIG DILEMMAS WITH TOXIC TREATMENTS

- http://www.dailymail.co.uk/health/article-2643751/Most-doctors-terminally-ill-AVOID-aggressive-treatments-chemotherapy-despite-recommending-patients.html

## DIET HAS A ROLE IN MY RECOVERY

- http://www.care2.com/causes/10-fermented-drinks-to-make-at-home.html#ixzz48LDRzMvo

## MONEY AND SOCIAL SECURITY

- Medicine prices 2015 - 2016 (prices in Finland, before government compensation)
- Asacol 400 (34,46 €/100 tablets)
- 6 tablets daily = 2,06 €
- 63,86 € / month / 31 days
- 766, 32 / year

- 7663,20 € / 10 years
- Pentasa 500 (42,26 €/100 tablets)
- 4 tablets daily = 1,69 €
- 52,39 € / month / 31 days
- 628,68 € / year
- 6286,80 € / 10 years
- Remicade 400 ml
- app. 3000 € / fusion
- Taken every other month, 6 x a year
- 18.000 € / year
- 180.000 € / 10 years
- Prednisone 40 mg (The use varies very much. Some people have to use it all the time, some only occasionally.)
- 36,91 € / 100
- On average three regimen 110 € / a year
- 1100 € / 10 years
- Humira
- 600 € / a shot. Lasts for two weeks.
- 144,000 € / 10 years
- http://laakehaku.apteekkariliitto.fi
- http://edition.cnn.com/2015/09/10/health/expensive-medications-value/
- Reumaliitto

## THE WAY WE LIVE TODAY

- http://www.telegraph.co.uk/health-fitness/nutrition/overeating-killing-us-cut-eat/
- http://www.thelancet.com/journals/lancet/article/PIIS0140-6736(17)32367-X/fulltext
- Environ Health Perspect; DOI:10.1289/ehp.1408660
- Effect of Organic Diet Intervention on Pesticide Exposures in Young Children Living in Low-Income Urban and Agricultural Communities.
- Asa Bradman,[1*] Lesliam Quirós-Alcalá,[1,2*] Rosemary Castorina,[1] Raul Aguilar Schall,[1] Jose Camacho,[1] Nina T. Holland,[1] Dana Boyd Barr,[3] and Brenda Eskenazi[1] - http://ehp.niehs.nih.gov/1408660/http://www.breakingtheviciouscycle.info/
- http://www.who.int/mediacentre/news/releases/2017/increase-childhood-obesity/en/

## EGYPT – THE MIRACLE OF VARIOUS ANTI-BACTERIA

- http://timesofindia.indiatimes.com/india/Clove-to-solve-clean-water-woes/articleshow/1211146.cms

## PERU – THE MOST MAGICAL PLACE IN SOUTH AMERICA

- https://healthimpactnews.com/2013/17-reasons-why-you-need-a-mango-every-day/
- http://www.takepart.com/article/2015/10/20/subway-antibiotic-free

## GREECE – THE LAND OF GODS AND GODDESSES

- http://www.livestrong.com/article/324634-is-feta-cheese-healthy/
- https://draxe.com/feta-cheese-nutrition/
- http://www.greek-oliveoil.net/health.htm
- http://www.bbcgoodfood.com/howto/guide/why-are-mediterranean-diets-so-healthy

HANDY ALL-AROUND TRAVEL TIPS

- http://umm.edu/health/medical/altmed/supplement/melatonin
- greenmedinfo.com
- https://wakeup-world.com/2018/03/20/five-food-medicines-that-could-quite-possibly-save-your-life/

EASY TRAVEL FOOD

- https://foodbabe.com/2014/06/27/healthy-airport-food/

1. MIND

- New International Version, http://biblehub.com/matthew/17-20.htm
- https://www.psychologytoday.com/blog/sapient-nature/201401/the-need-love

2. DETOX

- https://forvibranthealth.wordpress.com/2013/08/27/12-foods-to-avoid-during-your-detox-or-cleanse/
- http://www.optimalhealthnetwork.com
- http://www.enemabag.com/colon-cleanse-alternative/
- Optimal health network, Young Living members
- Department of Diagnostic Imaging, Northern General Hospital NHS Trust, Sheffield, UK.
- https://www.ncbi.nlm.nih.gov/pubmed/7551780
- https://www.ncbi.nlm.nih.gov/pmc/articles/PMC3990147/

3. INDIVIDUAL DIET – FIND THE LEAST HARMING FOOD FOR YOU

- http://pulse.seattlechildrens.org/novel-diet-therapy-helps-children-with-crohns-disease-and-ulcerative-colitis-reach-remission/
- Elimination diet
  http://www.mindbodygreen.com/0-12540/the-simple-elimination-diet-that-could-change-your-life-forever.html
  http://www.joybauer.com/ibs/how-food-affects-ibs/
  https://draxe.com/elimination-diet/
- Dr. Steven Gundry: Heart surgeon and author of "Dr. Gundry's Diet Evolution.
  http://energyatanyage.com/
- Dietary polyphenols may be associated with longevity: Study
  14-Oct-2013
  High dietary intake of polyphenols may be associated with up to a 30% reduction in mortality rates in older adults, according to new research that identifies urinary concentrations of polyphenols as a more accurate measure of intake.
- http://www.nutraingredients.com/Research/Dietary-polyphenols-may-be-associated-with-longevity-Study
  identification of the 100 richest dietary sources of polyphenols: an application of the Phenol-Explorer database.
  Pérez-Jiménez J1, Neveu V, Vos F, Scalbert A.
- Author information: Clermont Université, Université d'Auvergne, Unité de Nutrition Humaine, Saint-Genes-Champanelle, France. https://www.ncbi.nlm.nih.gov/pubmed/?term=identification+of+the+100+richest+dietary+sources+of+polyphenols
  https://www.mindbodygreen.com/0-17145/10-best-polyphenol-rich-superfoods-why-you-should-be-eating-them.html

## HEALTHY OILS

- https://www.oliveoiltimes.com/olive-oil-basics/greeks-leading-olive-oil-guzzlers/35304
- http://www.worldatlas.com/articles/countries-that-smoke-the-most-cigarettes.html
- http://www.who.int/mediacentre/news/releases/2017/increase-childhood-obesity/en/
- http://articles.mercola.com/sites/articles/archive/2014/08/31/trans-fat-saturated-fat.aspx
- http://www.telegraph.co.uk/news/health/news/11981884/Cooking-with-vegetable-oils-releases-toxic-cancer-causing-chemicals-say-experts.html

## SUPPLEMENTS

- http://www.telegraph.co.uk/lifestyle/wellbeing/6028408/Chlorella-the-superfood-that-helps-fight-disease.html
- https://chriskresser.com/how-too-much-omega-6-and-not-enough-omega-3-is-making-us-sick/
- https://authoritynutrition.com/optimize-omega-6-omega-3-ratio/
- http://www.omega-3.se/en/food.html
- http://drhyman.com/blog/2010/08/24/vitamin-d-why-you-are-probably-not-getting-enough/
- https://www.vitamindcouncil.org/about-vitamin-d/am-i-getting-too-much-vitamin-d/
- *) https://www.ncbi.nlm.nih.gov/pmc/articles/PMC3908963/
- 1Academy for Micronutrient Medicine; Essen, Germany
- 2Institute for Medical Information and Prevention; Wiesbaden, Germany
- 3Universitätsklinikum des Saarlandes; Homburg/Saar, Germany
- 4St. Anna Hospital, Medical Clinic I; Herne, Germany
- 5Boston University Medical Center; Boston, MA USA
- **https://www.ncbi.nlm.nih.gov/pubmed/22204435

## CANNABIS

- http://www.ncsl.org/research/health/state-medical-marijuana-laws.aspx

## ANOTHER APPROACH BY FUNCTIONAL MEDICINE

- functionalmedicine.org

www.ingramcontent.com/pod-product-compliance
Lightning Source LLC
Chambersburg PA
CBHW052136270326
41930CB00012B/2914